POST-TRAUMATIC STRESS DISORDER...
where the past controls today!

During his twenty-one years of service, Andrew Rae was on the front line of his state Police Force, confronting scenes that should be viewed only through the sterile screen of a television. Not only were these horrors seen daily but he touched, heard and smelt them. Then, one quiet morning free of the usual chaos and drama, Andrew suffered a breakdown. He was now forced to face his biggest fear and fight his bravest battle... with himself.

Based on real life events, **Beneath The Cap** delves into the tortured minds of three police officers who share a bond much stronger than the uniform they wear. The day about to confront them could be happening to any police officer, anywhere in the world

The story may shock and confront you ...but YOU DECIDE!

ABOUT THE AUTHOR

The Author was born, and grew up in the Hunter Valley of New South Wales in eastern Australia, During his school years, he was active in sports and music. After completion of his education, he took up accounting while studying for a Commerce degree at the University of Newcastle.

Andrew Rae joined the New South Wales Police Force, graduating from his training at the NSW Police Academy at Goulburn in 1986. For the next twenty-one years, he served in four major country cities where duties were variously as a General Duties Officer, Highway Patrol Officer or Scene of Crime Officer, attaining the rank of Senior Constable. In 2006, he was diagnosed as suffering from Post-Traumatic Stress Disorder and discharged a year later.

During his service, he earned the National Medal, one of the awards under the Australian honours system for individuals who serve or protect the community at the risk of their own death, injury or trauma. Other awards included the New South Wales Police Medal, 15 year and 20 year clasps to this medal and a Local Area Command Citation in recognition of his outstanding professionalism.

Since his discharge he has been self-employed. He and his wife of twenty-five years, have two adult children. Six years after his medical discharge, Andrew Rae still suffers the effects of PTSD.

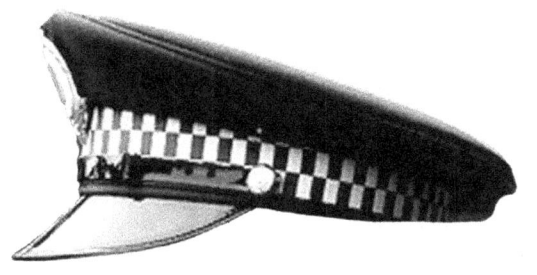

BENEATH
THE
CAP

ANDREW RAE

'*His mind and body were manipulated by a force he could not see, touch, hear or smell...*'
Post-Traumatic Stress Disorder. The past that controls today!

Published by
CUSTOM BOOK PUBLICATIONS
Second Edition

First Edition Custom Book Publications 2013

AUTHOR'S NOTE

Not in my wildest nightmares, of which I have had many, would I have thought it possible to be writing a dedication to a novel I have penned. Had it not been for the decision to join the New South Wales Police Force, my life today would be all the poorer for it.

To that end, I must thank the officers and staff I had the pleasure of working with over my twenty-one years. Your professionalism, dedication, mateship and good humour made the journey worthwhile.

To those officers still serving, I salute you in gratitude for the protection you provide our communities and pray for your protection so that you may return home safely at the end of each shift.

My wife has remained beside me, holding hands in support as I battled my demons. This commitment has shown your love more than words could ever say. Your tolerance and persistence has been instrumental in returning me to the man you married.

I am honoured to be called Dad by two of the best young adults anyone could find. Your passion for life bring a smile to my heart. Knowing my extended family was always there for me provided comfort. Your encouragement over a silly book idea provided motivation when it was lacking. Your proof reading and dubious opinions were appreciated.

Finally, to all who suffer Post-Traumatic Stress Disorder. *Live for today.*

> *'So do not be anxious about tomorrow,*
> *Tomorrow will look after itself.*
> *Each day has troubles enough of its own.'*
> Matthew 6:34

PROLOGUE

The man walked anxiously, his scuffed leather shoes a blur over the sand dusted pavement skirting the foreshore. Each crunching footfall was not of someone taking a leisurely stroll, but of someone's futile attempt to outpace his past.

His attire was somewhat dishevelled, the tail of his shirt hanging over the back of his trousers. With every other step, he would tug at the waistband to prevent them sliding down over his hips. Had his mind been in the present, he would have realised he had forgotten to fit the belt he normally wore. Getting dressed was somewhat of a challenge for the man these days. He did not know it yet, but his underpants were on inside out, and his shirt had buttons mismatched to their corresponding holes.

The three day stubble of beard covering his face only enhanced his haggard appearance. With a noticeable limp in his stride, the man appeared aged well beyond his years.

He lived an almost reclusive existence. His home had become the prison he used as protection from his insecurities and the vulnerability he felt in the outside world. Where possible, he avoided crowds and the suffocating chaos they created, leaving the safety of his self-imposed confinement only in the early hours of the morning. Protected by the comforting blanket that darkness provided, he left for work and completed his cleaning job by sunrise, so as to avoid the social contact inevitably following.

His surroundings were as distant to him as if they were occurring on the dark side of the moon. Oblivious to the barefoot children chased by the incoming swell, his eyes blinded by the shadow of memories.

His ears failed to register the crash of the waves, just the echoes of his padding feet that quickened to keep pace with each pounding heart beat throbbing in his head.

The salty sea air was lost to the breeze. Not even the sun warming his skin, could break through his tormented mind.

A couple strolling hand in hand approached. The man shied away, his head down to avoid any chance of their eyes meeting. Lungs strained as he held his breath before he darted off the footpath, crossing the narrow street to avoid their passing.

The nervous journey towards his eleven o'clock appointment suddenly came to a halt the instant the smell of butchered meat permeated his subconscious. The odour was a key, which unlocked a door deep within his mind. He turned and faced the butcher shop window, and gazed through his reflection at the choice meat cuts lining the display. His mouth turned dry as the sight triggered a nervous obsession. He began to knead his hands with such force it threatened to rub the skin raw.

The bright red door at the front of a multistorey building was now in view. Brass plates affixed to the brickwork, advertised the building's residents, but the man did not need to stop and read the level he required. Entering, he made his way to the stairwell and began to climb, one step at a time, his past silently following in each shoe impression left in the soft carpet.

*****

5.30AM

The sky brightened and turned powder blue, as the sun made its steady journey above the eastern horizon. At first, like a sprinter out of the blocks, it moved rapidly from its crouched position behind the mountains. Once free from their hold, the sun straightened, falling into a timeless rhythm towards the west.

Ricky became aware of his own cadence. It was not so much effortless, but more terminal and laboured. Each foot was thrown in front of the other as his ungainly jogging gait ate away at the miles. It may not have been pretty to look at, but each stride was taken with purpose and determination. Each thudding foot, with the accompanying grunt, was another step closer towards his future.

At just twenty-one, Ricky loved this time of day. He watched as the fashion parade of colour boldly strutted its stuff over the horizon, transforming the sky as spectacularly as any fireworks display. Through the strain of physical exertion, a smile broadened across his mouth and his brown eyes revelled in the spectacle.

Apart from marvelling at the dawn, Ricky also enjoyed this time of day watching a town awaken and come to life. Chifley was stirring, given life by those first warming rays. Located in the country about two and a half hours west of Sydney, just beyond the western slopes of the Blue Mountains, the town and its locals were starting another day's journey as well.

Ricky watched as a house light came on, a blind opened. He gave a quick wave to the milkman on his rounds.

He watched as cars pulled up in front of the newsagent, drivers dashing inside to buy their daily read. Chifley was stirring.

The rattle of the council garbage truck could be heard blocks away in the dawn quiet, a sound soon to be lost, mixed with a multitude of others as the day evolved.

'Come on son… keep it up, not far to go,' he panted to himself as he tried to ignore the throbbing of his thighs and the twinge in his shins.

Nearing his goal to jog five kilometres, he turned left into Browning Street and was thankful for the slight decline. He managed to quicken his pace a little, partly to try and finish with a spurt, but moreover to reduce the time he had to endure the pain he was inflicting upon himself.

Ricky ran past a middle aged man, well dressed in a suit and tie with a backpack held in one hand slung over his shoulder. He was about to open the driver's door of his car parked against the kerb, when Ricky jogged by.

'Morning mate,' Ricky said in between puffs as he passed.

The man acknowledged the greeting with a slight nod of the head and cursory wave of his free hand. Ricky had always had a natural curiosity in his nature. He could not help wondering who the person was? Where was he going? Where did he work and what did he do? To find answers, Ricky considered the type of car the gentleman was driving, the way he was dressed and the quality of the home he had exited but in the end, it was all guess work and assumptions. The old saying of *don't judge a book by its cover* was very true and Ricky reminded himself to apply this same philosophy to people. Over the last year, however, he found this harder and harder to do.

It was a consequence of *The Job* as police called it, a unique role within a community. As a policeman, Ricky's primary role was to maintain law and order as set out by numerous Regulations and Acts of Parliament which governed his every decision. Ricky soon learnt it is more than this. He had been called upon to be involved in all manner of events. If something happened in a community, and there is no specific organisation or government agency to deal with the situation, then the logical people to call were the police … they would know what to do.

It had not taken Ricky long to realise that the better you were at forming an accurate opinion of someone's character, before even a word was spoken, the better you were at your job. It could even assist in protecting yourself from harm, yet none of these internal opinions showed through the mask of authority and polite respect he displayed to the world. His physical reactions did nothing to reveal the constant re-

3

evaluation taking place in his mind. Ricky was certain of one thing though, his opinion never changed until a person displayed evidence to the contrary.

'Come on,' he grunted again as he made the final turn into Ennis Way and sprinted the final fifty metres to the front steps of his unit. With both hands, he grasped the handrail at the base of several steps leading to his front door. Bending his lean, muscular, one-hundred and eighty centimetre frame forward, he placed his head between his outstretched arms, forcing himself to remain on his feet, rather than collapse in an untidy mess on the ground. Water dripped from his shortly cropped brown hair that was darkened black with sweat. His mouth sucked in long deep breaths, fully inflating his lungs and then forced them back out noisily as he took the time to recover. He could feel blood pulsing through his body and hear it as it throbbed through his head. Ricky felt alive.

'Straighten and stay upright,' he told himself, recalling the advice of Physical Training instructors at the Police Academy.

'Slow and deep,' he told his breathing, willing compliance.

Jogging was something that Ricky did not really enjoy but he had not gotten out of the habit since leaving the academy. When he graduated, he vowed never to jog again but the conditioning and fitness level he achieved there was something he did not want to lose.

With the guilt he felt if he did not exercise daily added, he was motivated to keep pounding the pavement.

'This seemed so much easier at the academy,' he told himself as his breathing started to quieten and ease. Ricky smiled as he thought of those days. He knew it felt harder now, because he no longer had that horrible little man yelling in his ear. Physical Training Instructor Senior Constable Worthington thought motivation was best instilled by fear. His bellowing threatened all manner of physical harm and discomfort if you did not pick up the pace. The P.T. Instructor would even raise doubts about your parentage being the cause of your lack of physical excellence. This he managed to eloquently express in an impolite way… something about your mother having had carnal knowledge with a three-toed sloth.

Ricky started to climb his front steps and gave a little chuckle at the memory.

A voice came from behind. 'Morning, Ricky. You're in a good mood today.'

Ricky turned and saw his neighbour from the adjoining unit. 'Hi, Pete, just getting the day off to a good start,' he replied, turning on a step to look down.

'You should have told me you were going for a run,' Pete added seriously. 'I would have come with you.'

Ricky's mouth spread into a smirk. 'Really.'

Pete gave his stomach a flattening pat. 'Don't let this weathered exterior fool you. Below lays a well-balanced and oiled machine.'

Another laugh passed through Ricky's lips. 'And how many home brews does it take to keep that machine well oiled?'

Pete was in his mid-forties, had never married and did live a healthy and active lifestyle. He coached a local junior football team in the winter months and during summer he umpired first grade cricket. 'That brew lad, will keep me going till I'm a hundred,' he replied, trying unsuccessfully to keep a straight face.

'Where are you off to this early anyway?' Ricky enquired.

'I have to duck into Sydney for a couple of days with work,' Pete replied. 'What about you? Are you off today?'

Unlike most people, Ricky did not hate going to work yet. 'No. I start at seven. I've actually got a couple of day shifts in a row.'

'I've noticed you've been coming and going at all hours lately,' said Pete. 'I'm pleased it's not me doing all that shift work. It's a young person's game.'

'At least you don't get bored doing the same thing every day. Besides, it doesn't seem to worry me. I sleep really well whether it's night or during the day.'

'Ah, to be young again,' Pete lamented.

'Have a safe trip,' Ricky said, continuing to climb his front steps.

Pete gave a parting wave. 'Thanks.' He turned and walked towards his car.

Ricky opened his front door and entered the tiny, one bedroom unit. He heard himself repeating what he had just told Pete about not getting bored doing the same thing every day. His life today was far removed from the one he was living a little over eighteen months ago.

After leaving high school, Ricky found a full time job as a trainee accountant. Like most young people, he did not really know what he wanted to do with his life.

At one point, he considered leaving school early to become a cabinet maker, but then chose to continue with his education. After his Higher School Certificate, he applied for numerous jobs and just happened to snag the accountant one while he was still living at home with his parents. Ricky had been instilled with a strong work ethic from an early age. No one in his family, or anyone he knew, had been on welfare, so he knew nothing else other than to get up in the morning and go to work. Whether you enjoyed, or wanted to do it, was not relevant.

His job as a trainee accountant required him to work five days a week between the civilised hours of nine to five. He would then head off to university lectures three nights a week between six and nine in order to complete a Bachelor of Commerce Degree. They were long and boring days. Unable to yet afford a car, he spent forty-five minutes travelling each way on the train. Ricky would see the same unsmiling faces each morning on the platform and while on the train, those same faces would stare blankly out the carriage windows, watching the world pass in a blur. Some would bury their heads in a newspaper or book. The only sound was the clatter of steel wheels as they passed over every join in the line, the only movement the rhythmic sway of bodies, tossed around in unison as the train rocked and rolled from side to side.

Ricky had a fascination with people and would fill in his time on the trip by studying them, wondering how long they had been undertaking this daily ritual. He did not know it then, but the time would come when he would crave to have this routine back in his life – a life where he had control of his own daily outcome.

Once at his destination these same passengers, with their emotionless faces, became a single moving mass of humanity as they scuttled from the platform before being absorbed by the towering office blocks. Fortunately for Ricky, his work place was only one block from the station so he did not have far to scuttle. The building he worked in still had an old, manually operated elevator with no buttons to push to nominate your destination. No flashing lights to watch so you knew when you got there but this lift had something better.

It had Old *Charlie*. Charlie, in his seventies, was the lift driver. His tool of trade was the old stool with a cushion with more tape on it than vinyl. That was it – Charlie sat there all day and operated the lift with a worn, brass control handle. He knew everybody by name and on what floor they worked.

In the three years Ricky worked in the building, he had never known Charlie to miss a day sick.

Charlie considered himself to be a chauffeur, and all good chauffeurs wore a cap – his as worn as his stool, never straight but worn with pride. He was cheerful and engaging with a broad range of topics expressed eloquently so long as the conversation was before one. On his return from lunch he was as pissed as a sailor on shore leave. He sat slumped on his stool, his head tilted to the side, resting comfortably on the wall of the elevator. From then his only conversation consisted of a dribbling, unintelligible series of sounds followed by a laugh that shook his whole body. Even so, he managed to stop the elevator on the correct floor, without fail. Ricky could not help but think that this is what you become when you do the same thing day after day.

Ricky's own day was predictable and routine. The only variety in the work was the different client names that appeared on the books and accounts on which he was working, and this detail only mattered when it came to completing his six minute pad where he had to account for every six minutes of his day. It was then used to complete his time sheet for billings… exciting stuff.

University was just something he had to do because his accountancy job required it. For many students who attend university, it is all about living the uni life. He did not see it that way and struggled to achieve any solid results even though he had the academic ability to succeed. He simply lacked motivation and interest, not helped by his economics lecturer who would deliver lectures dressed only in a hessian bag as he was in *touch with the earth*.

Now effectively a full time student as he was unemployable outside the halls of academia. He preached on the economic workings of the world, but had never lived or done anything productive. Ricky could not stand him.

There was one subject at university that did spark Ricky's interest – he excelled in the law component of his studies making him consider a change in the direction of his life.

His first thought was to transfer over to a law degree and become a solicitor. Ricky quickly disregarded this option as he could not see it being much different to what he was now doing… and he could not see himself defending some scum bag in court for a crime they most likely committed. He was after excitement in his life. There was only one option. Going against all advice from family and friends, Ricky joined the police force.

Sweat was still soaking into his singlet top when Ricky walked into his bedroom. His radio was on. The voice of the news announcer caught his interest. Two words in particular snapped Ricky out of his daydream. 'Police pursuit.'

'Last night in the town of Appleton,' the news announcer said with precise diction. 'Two local males tried to evade capture by police after being disturbed breaking into the bottle shop. The men fled the scene in a stolen car they had used to smash the front window of the shop. The police pursuit of the offenders lasted for twenty minutes, ending when the stolen car lost control and collided with a tree. Although injured, two men were arrested by police at the scene.'

Ricky reached across his bed and turned the radio off, not interested in hearing the sport and weather reports. He stripped off his sweaty clothes and headed for the shower.

'I wish I had been working in Appleton last night,' he mumbled. 'I can't wait to be in a pursuit. I'll get to test out all that advanced driver training I did at the academy.'

6.00AM

'Daddy, daddy, you're on the TV,' shouted young Jordan as he ran up the hallway to his father's bedroom.

Little six year old Jordan jumped onto his father's bed, bubbling with excitement. 'Come quick daddy, you're on TV.'

'No I'm not,' Jordan's father Rowdy, replied sleepily. 'I'm in bed.'

'But you're on the TV too. Come see,' Jordan persisted as he bounced onto his father enthusiastically.

Rowdy's mouth gapped into a yawn. 'All right, I have to get up anyway. You're sure it's not just someone who looks like me?'

Jordan's excitement did not waiver. 'It's you daddy, it really is. Come an' see.'

Rowdy climbed out of bed slowly and put his two feet on the floor, then paused a moment. The willingness to rise further did not come easy. It was forced motivation to get up and face the new day. He rose with considerable effort and sighed. Jordan grasped his father's hand and began to run back towards the family room. He pulled Rowdy off balance. 'Hang on mate … your old man has to get all his parts moving first.'

Rowdy was only thirty-four years but no longer moved with the freedom of his youth. The joints in his legs and hips no longer responded quickly to his commands to move. They required some gentle coaxing into action. His tall, slim build no-longer as robust as it once had been. The faint lines emerging across his brow and tugging at the corners of his eyes, were starting to tell a life's story.

As he was led up the hallway by his son's hand, his daughter, Anne, emerged from her bedroom as they passed. She was still wiping the sleep from her eyes.

'Morning, squirt,' Rowdy said, stopping to give her a hug.

At nine, Anne had always been the smallest child in all her school classes, so Rowdy had affectionately nicknamed her *squirt*.

'Jordan said I'm on the TV,' Rowdy said as they parted. 'But I think he's seeing things.'

'No I'm not,' Jordan said with all the firmness his six years could muster. 'You come and see too, Anne.'

All three walked into the neat and tidy family room. Rowdy's wife, Emma, was already in the kitchen, busily preparing breakfast for the children and packing school lunch boxes. Like all mornings, she had turned the television on to catch the news.

Rowdy sat on the worn floral lounge facing the television while Anne and Jordan snuggled either side. Behind, Emma moved from one side of the kitchen to the other, opening cupboard doors, rattling pots and pans, flicking the kettle on to boil and dropping dirty utensils into the sink. She had been so busy she failed to notice the TV news item. She looked up and her movements slowed as she concentrated on the images flashing on the screen. She froze when she recognised her husband.

Ricky stood in front of the mirror and finished doing up the last button on his freshly starched and ironed police shirt. With a detailed eye he examined his reflection. He was proud of the job he was doing and made sure it showed in the uniform he wore. To Ricky, how you looked was a reflection on how you did your work. If you dressed like a slob, then that was probably a good indication of the care and dedication to which you undertook your work.

Ricky was no slob. Not in appearance, or his work. Like everyone, Ricky made mistakes and was not perfect but he did do his utmost not to make the same mistake twice.

As Ricky examined his uniform in the mirror, he noticed the button on his left breast pocket was upside down.

The button was made of metal and much larger than those which held his shirt together at the front. Emblazoned with a crown, which although ornamental, proved to be functional when attached to the flap of the pocket, rather than the pocket itself. This meant he could easily access the pocket without having to undo the button. As this pocket was used to house his official police notebook and pen, it received frequent use. Being one of the Queen's men, he showed his respect by straightening the button to its upright position.

Ricky checked that his metal identification number, 6034, was level above the pocket. Every time he looked at this number he could not help but do the maths. Added together they totalled thirteen, his birth date. He grinned. He viewed this as an omen that this was the career he was meant to be doing.

Satisfied that everything was in its rightful place and all shirt and trouser creases were like a knife edge, Ricky turned away from the mirror and thought about breakfast.

The glare of the television screen flickered from image to image. Amplified sounds filled his mind. Rowdy was no longer seated beside his children in the comfort and security of his home. His mind was transported back eight months when he was working a night shift as a Highway Patrol Senior Constable. It was two in the morning and Rowdy was driving his highway patrol vehicle on the Great North Highway through the rural township of Benstown.

'It's a nice quiet night so far,' commented Rowdy idly to his offsider Bryan. He drove across the curving concrete bridge that divided the town, and its twenty-five thousand citizens. Benstown had the wide but shallow Coal River flowing through its heart, the river providing the lifeblood that irrigators sourced to farm the rich alluvial floodplains surrounding the town. His offsider and observer for the shift lay comfortably reclined in the passenger seat.

'Yep, just the way I like it. Very few cars moving about and even fewer people,' Bryan replied. Bryan was a few years older than Rowdy but a couple of months junior within the service. Bryan worked his shoulders into the backrest of his seat as he got comfortable. He crossed his arms over his chest and closed his eyes as if to sleep.

'You know, Rowdy,' said Bryan. 'I think these night shifts aren't too bad. My wife can't nag me. The kids aren't around to whinge and whine. Life doesn't get much better really.'

'Yeah, it's just great if you've got a personal chauffeur to drive you around while you take a nap. Anyway, aren't you supposed to be my observer for the shift?'

'I am,' Bryan said, still with his eyes shut tightly. 'I'm just observing the back of my eyelids for a moment. I'm sure you will let me know if I see something else in the meantime.'

'How about I just let you know when it's seven-thirty and time to knock off,' Rowdy replied jokingly.

Bryan's mouth opened into a wide long yawn. 'Make sure you set the alarm then. I wouldn't like to be late knocking off.'

Rowdy had worked side by side with Bryan for too many years to think he was serious. He was happy for his colleague to make the most of a quiet period. 'Certainly sir,' Rowdy replied respectfully. 'Will there be anything else, sir? A hot chocolate perhaps?'

Bryan accented his voice with an aristocratic tone.

'Well, while you're at it, my good chap, be a good chauffeur and turn the radio up a bit. I quite like this song.'

Rowdy laughed as he leant forward across the steering wheel and turned up the volume on the commercial radio. 'Bad Moon Rising' filled the cabin of the highway patrol car. The dashboard clock clicked over to two-oh-one.

Rowdy drummed his fingers on the steering wheel in time with the music. As he approached the intersection with White Avenue, the police radio came to life.

'Bowen 20 urgent,' crackled a female voice from the radio's small speaker.

Bryan snapped upright from the passenger seat, his eyes wide awake. He quickly cut short the song by turning the commercial radio off. At the same time he turned the volume on the police radio up. Rowdy smiled at the speed his offsider had reacted; he had seen this instant reflex many times in the past when Bryan appeared oblivious to his surroundings. His eyes may have been closed, but all his other senses remained active and alert.

A high pitched tone then emanated from the radio. Lasting only seconds, the alert tone, activated by the Kingstown Police radio operator seventy kilometres away, was the signal for all other cars and stations to standby.

'All standby, Bowen 20 only,' said the calm voice of the male operator.

The small town of Bowen was located just twenty kilometres south of Benstown. Bowen 20 was the call sign of the police vehicle attached to the two-man police station there. The vehicle was a fully marked, dual cabin, with a prisoner cage mounted behind. The vehicle was not built for speed nor had it nimble handling qualities.

'Bowen 20. I'm in pursuit of an ambulance,' the female driver replied over the sound of her vehicle's siren.

'Bowen 20, your location, direction and speed?' asked the radio operator with an even tone in his voice.

Bowen 20 replied with a sharp voice that increased in pitch and told of her nervousness. 'Radio, I'm currently heading north on the Great North Highway.'

Silence then filled the airway as the radio operator waited for the driver of Bowen 20 to finish relaying the information he had requested. None came.

'Location and speed Bowen 20?' asked the radio operator again.

The female officer's voice had now reached yelling pitch. 'Just crossing White Creek, north of Bowen, doing one-hundred and thirty.'

The radio operator was an experienced man. He knew a common mistake police made in pursuits was to give their own speed rather than that of the offending vehicle.

'Speed of the offending vehicle Bowen 20?' prompted the operator.

The female officer still yelled, adrenalin surging through her body. 'It's pulling away from me like I'm standing still. It's got to be doing one-fifty plus.'

Bowen Police Station was staffed by two officers, and Rowdy knew that Bowen 20 was currently being driven by Constable First Class Sheerwood. Dawn had been in the job about six years and her inexperience was obvious through the radio.

Realising the situation to come, Rowdy and Bryan gave each other a knowing look. They did not have to say a word. They had been in this situation countless times before. Rowdy put his right blinker on and casually made a U-turn. The big V8 motor roared as Rowdy pressed the accelerator pedal effortlessly to the floor and sent it rocketing south towards Bowen. 'Looks like we're up to bat,' said Bryan softly.

Bryan leant forward and activated the lights and sirens on the highway patrol car. He was then pushed back into his seat again by the force of the vehicle's rapid acceleration. His rest was over.

The radio operator continued. 'Bowen 20, category of vehicle and driver certification?'

Dawn's voice now noticeably quivered. Her nerves were causing her to forget her training and replied, 'Radio, I'm in a Rodeo caged truck.'

All police vehicles were categorised from one to four as to their suitability to engage in pursuits – one, the most suitable; four the least. The type of vehicle, its build, configuration and whether it is fully, partially or unmarked, were all taken into account when a vehicle was categorised. Dawn's vehicle was a category three, and whilst it was not the best vehicle to pursue in, it still could be used if no other higher category vehicle was available.

'Your licence certification, Bowen 20?' asked the radio operator.

'Bronze, radio,' replied Dawn with an excited high pitched yell.

All constables who graduate from the police academy after having passed their driving course are Bronze Certified. As they undertake further advanced driver training and pass assessments, an officer can progress to Silver and then Gold Certification. This is an easy method of gauging an officer's driving ability.

'I bet the DOI has now had to put his newspaper down,' Bryan said to Rowdy.

'Yes, he may even have to get up off his comfortable chair,' replied Rowdy as he again crossed Benstown Bridge, this time at high speed.

The Police Radio Operations Room is tucked away in a small, windowless office on the third floor of Kingstown Police Station. It controls all police communications from the Central Coast to the Queensland border by both civilian public servants and sworn police officers and hardly ever have a quiet night. Overseeing the operation is the Duty Operations Inspector or DOI. He has the authority to make numerous decisions affecting day to day policing before having to proceed to the next level of authority.

One area the DOI closely monitors is police pursuits and whether or not he should let them proceed or order they be terminated.

'Do you reckon the DOI will terminate?' Bryan asked Rowdy.

Rowdy did not reply immediately as he contemplated the situation. 'The only thing in our favour is that there is hardly another soul on the road tonight. We haven't passed a car in the last fifteen minutes. I can only assume it's the same down at Bowen.'

'I don't think Dawn will be instilling the DOI with much confidence at the moment,' stated Bryan. 'The information that should only take seconds to relay is getting drawn out a bit.'

Rowdy glanced down between the spokes of the steering wheel and watched the white needle on the illuminated speedometer pass one-hundred and thirty kilometres an hour. His heart rate felt just as quick. 'Yes and it's not finished yet,' he said, consciously fighting to remain calm and alert while his own adrenaline began rushing through his veins.

Rowdy was aware of the hazards of tunnel vision which can affect even the most experienced officers. He kept his eyes moving, moving them from side to side, as he tried to take in everything around him.

'The original offence, Bowen 20?' asked the radio operator.

Dawn yelled her reply over the wailing sirens. 'The ambulance has been stolen, radio.'

The radio operator again had to prompt for basic information. 'Weather, road and traffic conditions, Bowen 20.'

'No other cars in sight,' shrieked Dawn. 'It's fine and the road is sealed and dry.'

'Shit,' Rowdy exclaimed as he jumped hard on the brakes. His car dipped its nose instantly as the vehicle slowed rapidly. Bryan felt his chest press against the seat belt.

'That's an understatement,' Bryan said as he placed his eyeballs back into their sockets.

Looming out of the darkness in front of them, the roadway was a mass of moving people. The drunken patrons, from the Queens Hotel streamed out through the front doors of the establishment and onto the roadway as the late closing time was enforced by security staff.

The mass of people were oblivious to the flashing blue and red lights that danced from building to building. The wail of the siren was lost in the drunken uproar as the rabble made its way across the highway, where they attempted to gain access to the Kings Hotel whose closing time was not for another two hours – four am.

'It never ceases to amaze me how these idiots still think we're a taxi,' said Bryan shaking his head. Drunks barely capable of standing, attempted to wave them down whilst shouting to hail what they thought was a cab.

'Get out of the fucking way, you morons,' Bryan shouted from inside the cabin towards the humanity stumbling across the highway.

Rowdy continued to slow his vehicle and alternated his siren between the yelp and wail function by pushing the steering wheel horn. The crowd of drunken revellers made no attempt to provide a passage. 'I don't think they heard you, Bryan.'

With no one in the crowd possessing enough functioning brain cells to make a conscious decision, Rowdy assumed some primitive survival sense must have kicked in as those closest to the approaching vehicle slowly began to part.

'Is your window fully up mate?' Rowdy asked Bryan without taking his eyes off the boiling crowd in front of him. At the same time, his finger located the electric window switch fitted to his door trim and toggled it up to make sure.

'Yeah, why?'

'I've already showered today. I don't want to have another one,' replied Rowdy as Bryan glanced across at him, his face reflecting his confusion. Rowdy was concentrating too hard on the crowd to explain himself further.

Barely moving, the police vehicle entered the parting crowd and made steady progress. Bodies swarmed around it as fluid as water. Hands shot from the surrounding horde and rocked its journey like the sway of a ship at sea. The whole time, a gale of sound buffeted the car as drunks mouthed muffled words they did not believe to be compliments.

Rowdy steered his way through the tail end of the mob. A face suddenly appeared close to Bryan's window and spat onto the closed glass. No sooner had the chunky yellow saliva started to trickle down its surface and the face was lost back into the crowd.

'I don't think they like you, Bryan,' said Rowdy to his furious offsider.

Bryan swivelled in his seat and looked behind into the crowd. 'That dirty, rotten, filthy bastard,' he said with real hatred in his voice. 'That's one face I'm not going to forget.'

Rowdy knew full well Bryan had the memory of an elephant. If it was a week, a year or even two, Rowdy was confident Bryan and the spitter would meet again.

Rowdy exited the crowd and again pressed the accelerator pedal to the floor. The thumping V8 echoed down the highway as he continued the journey south.

'Current location and speed, Bowen 20,' enquired the radio operator.

'Still northbound on the Great North Highway, near Bell Road. The ambulance is under lights and sirens about one kilometre ahead of me, still doing one-fifty plus,' replied Dawn. A measure of calmness had re-entered her voice, now that the ambulance had extended its lead.

The radio operator still dug for information. 'Number of persons on board the offending vehicle, Bowen 20?'

'Only one, radio.'

Satisfied with the information that he now had the radio operator again sounded the alert tone. 'Standing by for any vehicle in the vicinity to assist Bowen 20, currently in pursuit of a stolen ambulance, one kilometre north of Bell's Road on the Great North Highway.'

Bryan had been expecting the request and lifted the radio handpiece to his mouth.

'Benstown 202, radio,' said Bryan calmly giving their vehicle's call sign.

'Benstown 202 only, go ahead,' replied the radio operator.

The stolen ambulance was still ten kilometres away from their location when Bryan continued. 'Radio, we're currently south on the Great North Highway in Benstown, crossing Gould Street. We will take over as the primary pursuit vehicle when in range. Category 1 vehicle. Gold driver and observer. For your information, we just passed a large group of inebriated hotel patrons spilling onto the roadway between the Queens and Kings Hotels. They will cause a public safety problem if this ambulance continues at speed.'

Bryan was cautious with his words. Everything he said was being recorded in the radio operations room. The recording would be kept and archived to be used in any future court proceeding or internal police inquiry.

'What happened to, *the dirty rotten filthy bastards* we just passed?' Rowdy enquired.

'They still are, and we should have run over one of them just to set an example to the others,' lamented Bryan.

Rowdy continued at speed under emergency lights and sirens.

'Bowen 20, keep your location coming,' prompted the radio operator.

'Still northbound on the Great North Highway. Just approaching the Mitchell Road intersection,' replied Dawn in an almost normal voice. 'I've lost sight of the ambulance. I can only assume it's still heading back to Brookstone.'

This was the first indication that Dawn knew more about the circumstances surrounding the stolen ambulance. Had she passed on her knowledge to the radio operations centre then the DOI may not have allowed the pursuit to continue.

Earlier, Dawn was patrolling in Bowen when she observed an ambulance travelling south on the highway. She watched as it swerved sharply to its left and then came to a sudden stop. The driver's door flew open at the same time, quickly followed by a stumbling ambulance officer who staggered away from the vehicle. No sooner was the officer clear of the ambulance; it accelerated into a harsh U-turn. Smoke billowed from the rear tyres as rubber peeled off onto the road. In a blaze of red light from its emergency beacons, the ambulance powered on, back in the direction it had just come.

Dawn had approached the stranded ambulance officer. He told her he had been escorting a psychiatric patient from Brookstone, which was the next major town located forty-five kilometres north of Benstown. He was conveying the patient to a hospital in Kingstown and as he was not a violent patient, or in need of physical medical treatment in transit, he was the single ambulance officer rostered to perform the escort.

As the ambulance neared the township of Bowen, the male patient started to ask for certain sexual favours to be provided. The patient became agitated after having his advances refused. He then attempted to physically fondle the ambulance driver who became fearful for his safety and made the decision to abandon ship. In his haste to distance himself from the patient, the officer did not turn the motor of his vehicle off and left the keys in the ignition.

The psychiatric patient then took full advantage of the opportunity and chose to drive himself home.

Rowdy heard Dawn give her last location. Up ahead, some two kilometres in the distance, Rowdy could see the revolving flash of red light of the ambulance approaching. Rowdy began to slow his highway patrol car.

'No point us continuing on and pass each other going in the opposite direction,' Rowdy said to Bryan. 'I'll let him come to me.'

Bryan raised the radio handpiece that was permanently affixed to the palm of his right hand.

'Benstown 202, radio. We have the ambulance in sight. It has continued north past Mitchell Road.'

Rowdy made a leisurely U-turn and stopped in the breakdown lane facing north. His lights and sirens were still activated and pierced through the night.

'Are you in pursuit Benstown 202?' asked the radio operator.

Bryan's voice continued to be level, hiding the excitement that filled him within. 'Not at this stage, radio. We are stopped waiting for the ambulance to pass us at Dark Creek, opposite the old Witham Homestead.'

Rowdy watched in his rear vision mirror as the ambulance approached at high speed. When about three hundred metres behind, Rowdy pushed the accelerator of his pursuit car to the floor once more. The bonnet rose in front of him. Roaring ferociously, all the vehicle's power gripped the road and shot forward. The car jerked with each gear change as Rowdy, still in the breakdown lane, accelerated as fast as possible.

The patrol car rocked from the air turbulence as the speeding ambulance passed.

'Shit, he's got it wound up,' Bryan remarked.

Rowdy watched as his speedometer needle passed one hundred and sixty kilometres an hour.

'He does seem to be in a bit of a hurry,' Rowdy added as he merged back into the northbound lane, as the transmission shifted into top gear.

'Benstown 202 in pursuit,' Bryan said down the radio handpiece and then continued in the same steady voice. 'Northbound. Great North Highway Witham, approaching Range Road. Speed one-eighty. Traffic light. Single lane carriageway. Dry bitumen. Weather fine. Rural area sparsely populated.'

Bryan relayed the information concisely, in a matter of seconds, what had taken Dawn minutes and then after considerable prompting.

'Standby Benstown 202, we're getting some information through from ambulance control,' said the radio operator hesitantly.

'202 copy. Crossing Little Baker Bridge, still one-eighty.'

At one-hundred and eighty kilometres an hour, Rowdy was as alert as any person could be. All his senses were in a heightened state as adrenaline continued to surge through his body. At this speed, Rowdy was covering fifty metres every second and there was no room for errors. Any sudden movement of the steering wheel or a touch of the brakes at the wrong time could spell disaster for the two officers.

'Easy does it son,' Rowdy said to relax himself. 'Fast and smooth. Breathe slowly and pick your lines.'

Rowdy took control of both his body and the car. The second of the two small creek crossings approached. The rough black tar shining under the headlights disappeared under the vehicle in a smooth blur.

'Crossing Big Baker Bridge. Still one-eighty. Same conditions,' said Bryan to give a quick update.

Rowdy kept a gap of two seconds between his vehicle and the ambulance. With an average reaction time of one second, this left Rowdy with a one second buffer zone or fifty metres to avoid anything that happened ahead of them.

Rowdy had travelled this section of road countless times. He knew every corner, bump and pothole. Although he could not see it yet through the darkness, he knew the ambulance was approaching a left bend about three hundred metres away. At first, the bend seems to sweep gently to the left, but then becomes deceivingly sharper as you enter the curve.

'Benstown 202, from the DOI, you are instructed to terminate. 202 terminate the pursuit,' said the calm voice of the radio operator over the airway.

The Duty Operations Inspector had been in contact with the ambulance control centre and was informed of the circumstances of the ambulance being stolen. As the identity of the offender was known, the likely location he was heading to and the speeds involved, the DOI made the wise and informed decision to terminate.

Just as the radio operator had begun his message to terminate the pursuit, Rowdy saw the glow of brake lights from the rear of the ambulance glare across his windscreen.

Dread filled Rowdy's voice. 'Oh no.'

The driver of the stolen ambulance had seen the corner sharpen and braked heavily, causing a weight transfer from the back of the vehicle to the front. The tyres lost traction as the rear of the ambulance started to slide to the right. The driver made the mistake of turning harder to the left.

Rowdy and Bryan watched on helplessly. Time seemed to stop. The footage they were watching through their windscreen played frame by frame. He could not help but raise his usually quiet voice. 'He's lost it,' he shouted. Rowdy lifted his accelerator foot slowly, not wanting to make the same mistake as the driver of the ambulance.

In a reflex movement, Bryan clutched the grab handle mounted on the roof lining above his door with his left hand. 'Christ no,' he blurted loudly. Bryan was unable to mask the genuine fear in his voice as the tragedy before him unfolded. 'He's headed for that farm house.'

The driver of the ambulance had lost all control over his vehicle. It continued to slew to the right as the laws of physics took over. Powerless to do anything to prevent the tragedy, Rowdy and Bryan could only watch on as the ambulance exited the apex of the corner. It crossed to the wrong side of the road, continuing its journey towards the farmhouse. Unusual for this rural area, the house was only metres away from the road's edge.

The house was a modest dairy farmer's cottage, clad with timber and a corrugated iron roof. It had the appearance of a story book drawing with its front door in the centre and a window either side. Neat flower beds surrounded its footings, and a brick chimney rose from the ground on one side. The front of the cottage was protected from the elements by a timber post veranda. Two brick steps led onto the deck in line with the door.

Inside the house a young family was asleep. The mother and father were in the bedroom to the left of the front door while their two children slept soundly in the bedroom on the right – all oblivious to the carnage heading their way.

The rear right side of the ambulance struck the leading edge of the veranda. Fortunately, the half metre high veranda prevented the ambulance from continuing on to plough through the front rooms. The ambulance slammed its way along the front of the veranda at one-hundred and eighty kilometres an hour, snapping all six hardwood roof posts like they were twigs. The iron roof sagged without its supports and was torn away from its mountings on the house.

The sudden cataclysm remodelling the front of the house woke all inside. Disorientated from sleep, the family had no idea what was the cause. The bedrooms shook violently and a deep rumble reverberated through the framework. It was like an earthquake had struck. Adding to the confusion, flashes of red light pierced the windows, illuminating the rooms in a devilish glow.

Over the splintering of timber, a satanic scream was heard as the siren of the ambulance filled the rooms.

The ambulance continued its path of destruction all the way to the opposite end of the veranda. The vehicle's speed had only been slowed marginally by the impact. It continued on through a steel farm gate located three metres past the house. The gate was torn from its hinges and wrapped around the front of the ambulance as it continued unimpeded into a grazing paddock.

Rowdy continued to slow his police vehicle. In a controlled manoeuvre, he crossed onto the wrong side of the road into the southbound breakdown lane and approached the crumbling house.

Bryan's lips parted against the microphone, but were unable to utter a word as he was blinded by a flash of light.

Rowdy raised a hand to shield his eyes from the searing glare. 'I can't see a thing,' he cried.

'Either can I,' Bryan yelled back, attempting to shield his own eyes. 'Just don't hit anything in the meantime.'

Neither officer heard the shattering of glass that came soon after the blinding flash. Rowdy's eyes adjusted from the burning blaze of light but found his vision blurred – not from the searing light, but from the shattered windscreen on his vehicle. Something had struck the windscreen directly in line with his head, fortunately not penetrating and continuing through.

The ambulance continued along its destructive path into the grazing paddock for another ten metres before it struck an old eucalypt iron bark stump. Felled years ago, and cut off at waist height, its girth measured two metres. The mighty tree stump was more than a match for the out of control ambulance. The front grill of the ambulance, still with the farm gate in place, disintegrated on impact. The ambulance's momentum continued forward, taking the vehicle up and over the massive hardwood. The rear of the ambulance catapulted into the air, taking down the power line feeding into the farm house. Sparks showered the somersaulting ambulance. Its engine ripped free and continued its own journey into the darkness beyond. High pressure fuel sprayed from severed lines and the ruptured fuel tank bathed everything around it, instantly ignited by falling sparks. A massive explosion erupted twenty metres into the night sky. It was as if the sun had been turned on by a switch. Blinding light turned the scene into day. A billowing mushroom cloud of flames and smoke leapt towards the stars.

As quickly as the explosion came, it was gone. The fuel swiftly burnt off and darkness consumed the scene again. The ambulance was left unrecognisable on its crumpled roof. Its undercarriage exposed to the heavens.

Rowdy quickly located the toggle switch to wind down his side window. He thrust his head through the opening and brought his highway patrol car to a stop outside the carnage of the farm house. He quickly assessed the scene before him.

'Get the fire extinguisher,' he said with urgency, Bryan left the vehicle with a swiftness that belied his size to retrieve the extinguisher from the boot. Rowdy leant across and opened the passenger glove box and pushed the boot release button. The radio handpiece lay on the passenger floor where Bryan had dropped it. Rowdy grabbed the coiled lead attached to it and sprung it back towards him.

'Benstown 202 radio,' Rowdy said with effort. 'The ambulance has lost control and collided with a house. I need ambulance, ambulance rescue and fire brigade to three-hundred metres north of our last location. Condition of driver or other persons unknown.'

Rowdy did not wait for the radio operator to reply. He ran from his vehicle over to the upturned and smoking ambulance. Bryan had just finished extinguishing the last of the flames. Neither Bryan nor Rowdy realised that in their haste, they had run over live power lines. Their focus was on finding the driver.

The patient capsule mounted on the ambulance was surprisingly intact. Its contents however, were a jumbled mess. Half its contents had littered the paddock when the rear doors were sprung open on impact with the ground. The rest of the vehicle was a mangled mess of steel and plastic. The front of the ambulance had been pushed back into the dashboard, surely trapping and maiming any person in their seat. Wheels were missing and the drive shaft buckled upwards.

Rowdy ran around the ambulance, stopping to peer through shattered window openings as he went. Bryan did the same but in the opposite direction. 'Where the bloody hell is he?' Bryan yelled.

Rowdy completed a second frantic lap around the ambulance. 'I can't see anyone,' he said with confusion. 'I'll check inside.'

Rowdy climbed through the open rear doors and walked along the capsule's roof. He straddled over equipment that now littered its once clean lines. Miraculously, the collapsible trolley bed remained securely fixed in place above his head. Rowdy stuck his head into what was left of the driver's cabin. 'There's nobody in here,' he yelled out to Bryan as he surveyed the crumpled cabin. 'If they were, they wouldn't be coming out in one piece.'

Rowdy made his way back out. His attention was immediately drawn past Bryan who met him as he climbed out of the shell. Rowdy looked back towards the farm house. A shape was silhouetted amongst the rubble of the half collapsed veranda. Rowdy was again forced to shield his eyes, this time from the glare of his vehicle's headlights that streaked across the scene. The red and blue emergency beacons atop his vehicle added to the confusing shadows as they danced across the house. He initially doubted what his eyes were seeing. It must be just a shadow caste from all the lights amongst the debris. Then he was sure of it.

'How the hell did he get back there?' said Rowdy in amazement and lowered his hand from above his eyes. Bryan, who thought Rowdy had been giving him a strange look, turned around to see the outline of a man sitting on the edge of the crumpled veranda deck. His head bowed down between his knees.

Rowdy's amazement turned to joy. 'He's okay. He got out okay.'

It seemed impossible that the driver of the ambulance could be the person sitting on the veranda, but in Rowdy's wishful mind it could not be anyone else.

Rowdy took several slow steps towards the forlorn man sagged on the veranda. Then, from behind, somewhere out of the darkness came a prolonged and gargled moan. Rowdy stopped and turned back towards Bryan. 'What was that?' he asked.

'Sounded like a cow to me,' Bryan replied as he turned and peered into the bleakness.

Both men starred into the darkness, tilting their heads sideways and straining their ears to pick up every little sound.

'There it is again,' Rowdy exclaimed and pointed. 'It's coming from that direction.'

The two officers ran into the gloom away from the ambulance, deeper into the paddock. Fifteen metres away they came across the prone body of a man lying still in the grass. Without any movement of his lips he let out another throaty moan. Unable to move, Rowdy was overcome by that soul wrenching feeling of being utterly helpless.

'He's alive.' Rowdy blurted out the obvious to break free from his own trance like state.

'He's not looking too good though.'

Rowdy became a police officer again. 'Go and update radio. See how far away the ambos are,' he snapped to Bryan.

When the ambulance struck the tree stump, its kinetic energy was reduced to nearly zero in a matter of seconds. Although the ambulance itself had come to a stop, everything not tied down inside kept moving. The same force projected the driver through the front windscreen at a speed of nearly one-hundred and sixty kilometres an hour.

Rowdy had to do something to try and help the man, even though the body before him was beyond anything that his training could assist. He ran through his first aid mantra – DRABC

Danger had certainly passed.

The man was moaning which was some sort of *Response*.

Airway. 'I need to check his airway,' Rowdy thought to himself. 'Jesus,' he continued to himself. 'The guy just attempted supersonic flight without a plane. Every bone in his body must be broken and his internal organs must be like scrambled eggs.'

Rowdy made the decision not to move him.

Breathing. His chest was rising and falling with the audible sound of his breathing as his lungs strained to function.

Circulation. There was a pulse in the man's wrist.

With his first aid ability all but exhausted, the only other thing he could do was check for external injuries and blood loss. Where to start? The man's face was covered in blood from numerous cuts but none appeared to be noticeably flowing. Rowdy scanned the man's clothing. Nothing appeared to be soaking through.

Rowdy again made the decision that the best course of action was to do nothing but monitor the unconscious man. There was nothing he could do that would have an effect on saving the man's life. 'Where's a bloody ambulance when you need one?' he jokingly said aloud to himself and looked back along the path of destruction to the farm house.

Within minutes, the quietness that had again returned to the tranquil rural setting turned into a scene of loud and urgent activity. Two ambulances, ambulance rescue truck and two fire tankers were at the scene. Dawn Sheerwood in Bowen 20 arrived along with two other police vehicles.

One was the Benstown General Duties truck crew and the other a detective's vehicle that was working a rare late shift in the area. Even the energy company that supplied and serviced the power lines to the town had an emergency crew on the way.

Night was turned into day as generators were fired up to provide lighting. All the emergency vehicles turned on the external speaker system fitted to their vehicle's radio. Nine vehicles lined the roadway, parked at various angles, and all with emergency lights flashing. Red, blue, and orange blended together to caste a carnival glow across the scene.

Three ambulance personnel frantically worked on the injured man. All his clothing had been cut away. He lay naked, making it easier to work and locate injuries.

Rowdy held an oxygen mask over the man's face after swabbing away thick, black and congealing blood. Below all the gore was a swollen, lacerated and bruised remnant of a face. The injured man lay semi-conscious as he was worked on. He gurgled as he breathed a mixture of air and blood into the oxygen mask. Whenever moved he would let out a high pitched howl of pain that only his subconscious felt. It was a howl that could be heard over all the noise of generators, shouts for more equipment and amplified radio messages. It was a howl that brought a chill to all that heard it.

Bryan stood to one side of the injured man holding an IV drip. With every anguishing howl, Bryan would look away and begin to whistle towards the night sky. Being at home with his nagging wife and whinging kids did not seem that bad a place to be right now.

The ambulance officers were preparing to encase the man's legs and lower torso with an inflatable pressure suit. This would assist to immobilise his legs, pelvis and lower spine which all had multiple fractures. The only clothing that he still wore were his shoes and socks. An ambulance officer removed these items from his left foot.

The front half of his foot flopped to the ground, completely severed through to the skin on the sole of his foot. Quickly grabbing the dangling toes, the officer pushed it back to its rightful place and exerted pressure to stem the fresh blood flow that soaked the ground. The foot was bandaged tightly and the inflatable pressure suit fitted.

The ambulance officers had done all they could to stabilise the injured man's condition. Just as they were placing him onto a spinal board, the air around them began to beat and throb. Faintly at first but then increasing in pitch as the rescue helicopter approached and prepared for its landing.

Everyone turned their heads and closed their eyes to protect themselves from the barrage of grass and dirt that pummelled their bodies. Those who were standing were forced to lean into the downdraught to prevent from being blown across the paddock.

The forward facing, night-sun spotlight lit the turbulent ground below as it swivelled on its axis three-hundred and sixty degrees in its search for power lines or other hazards it may encounter on its descent.

Safely on the ground, the helicopter powered down, its rotor blades sagging as the powerful motor whined to a stop. The crew of paramedics took over the care of the injured man who was soon loaded on board.

Within minutes, the helicopter disappeared back into the darkness. The beat of its rotors fading, and the flash of its navigation lights mingled with the stars.

Rowdy examined the scene around him. He looked past the wreckage to see Dawn leaning down with a hand on the shoulder of the distraught husband and father he had mistaken for the driver of the ambulance. He was still sitting on what was left of his front veranda. An electrician was at the top of a power pole. Firemen were coiling their hoses and stowing their extinguishers. Police sprayed white paint to mark the location and position of Rowdy's highway patrol vehicle along with the other objects from the ambulance that littered the paddock in preparation for the Police Crash Investigation Unit.

Rowdy couldn't help but think that this was his entire fault. He constantly replayed the event in his mind, looking for that point where all this could have been avoided.

'Hey, Rowdy, guess what I was just told,' Bryan yelled as he walked towards him.

'I've got no idea, Bryan,' Rowdy replied vacantly, still lost in his thoughts.

'It turns out this bloke was a psych patient and started to get frisky with the ambo,' Bryan continued to yell as he came closer.

Rowdy suddenly realised he did not even know the name of this *bloke* who was now fighting for his life. 'It may have helped to know that before we started the pursuit.'

'I suppose so… Anyway, if the ambo had just closed his eyes and thought of England and taken one for the team, none of this would have happened,' Bryan laughed.

Rowdy could not even force a smile to his face. He pointed over Bryan's shoulder in the direction of the farmhouse and said, 'It could have been worse.' Bryan turned and saw the farmer's wife walk out onto her remodelled veranda, clutching two young children in her arms.

The Duty Officer for the area, Inspector Barry Gosling arrived at the scene and called Rowdy and Bryan over. 'I should have known better than to let you pair play together,' he said.

'Sorry boss, but Rowdy led me astray again.'

Ignoring Bryan's comment, Inspector Gosling turned serious. 'I have to instruct you pair to no longer engage in any further conversation with each other. I just got word through that the offender died in flight. This is now being investigated as a death in police custody.'

Bryan's normally jovial face paled to a sullen expression. Perspiration streamed from his body and quickly soaked through his shirt. 'I need a cigarette,' was his verbal response to the news.

'Are you alright?' Emma asked. She stood behind her husband and placed a gentle hand on his shoulder. Rowdy still sat on the lounge in front of the television. His two children had lost interest in the news item and were giggling amongst themselves at the breakfast table.

Brought back into the present by his wife's touch, he reached up and clutched her hand and replied, 'Yeah, everything is fine.'

The television news presenter concluded by saying, 'Late yesterday the Coroner gave his report into the police pursuit and cleared police involved of any contributing negligence.' He went on to state, '…all police pursuit guidelines had been followed. A review, however, would be undertaken into the state ambulance service procedures for escorting psychiatric patients.'

'That's a relief,' said Emma, patting Rowdy's shoulder.

'Yeah, a long eight months compared to the time the pursuit lasted,' he replied. From the start of the pursuit to its fatal end was a distance of two thousand eight hundred metres. It had consumed fifty-six seconds of his life.

'You know love,' Rowdy said as Emma snuggled beside him on the lounge. 'It's fitting to hear of the Coronial Inquest result on the news and not from the Police Service.'

'Why's that?' inquired Emma.

'Within twenty-four hours of that pursuit I had heard from every local and regional newspaper, and radio station, as well as each of the national TV networks. Even international media groups were interested in the story. To this very day I still haven't been contacted by the Police Welfare Branch or had a debrief.'

Emma gave a consoling hug. 'You of all people should know by now that you're just a number in a big organisation.'

'Yeah, I know. Speaking of doing his job, I'd better get going. I start in under an hour.'

Rowdy had fourteen years' service under his belt and had spent the last five stationed at Benstown. Like all police, he started out performing general duties but transferred over to highway patrol after three years, although it was not the highway patrol role that attracted him to the job. Rather, it was the means of obtaining a transfer closer to where his extended family lived and where he wanted to settle down and start a family with Emma. He was not your stereotypical highway patrolman who liked the roar and power of a V8 motor, driving fast and imagining he was to be the next world champion. He was more the type who preferred to put his Volvo drivers cap on and sedately drive at ten kilometres under the speed limit.

On those rare occasions when he did lift the bonnet of a car to expose the motor, he would simply say, 'Well, would you look at that,' then close the bonnet in complete ignorance to its torque, kilowatt power, horse power or any other power that it was capable of producing. What he did know, was that if he was in the driver's seat and pushed the pedal on the right, the car moved. It stopped when he pushed the pedal on the left. The circular thing protruding from the dash he found very useful to avoid hitting anything else moving or stationary.

He was, however, more than capable of controlling a car at high speed when called upon. The advanced driver training and skid pan work he had performed over the past fourteen years was not wasted. Like everything Rowdy did, he liked to do it well and master it. He simply chose not to drive fast because he saw the inherent danger of it. He had been in the job too long and had attended hundreds of accidents. He realised it could happen to him one day, so he did his best to lengthen the odds.

It was said that Rowdy did not have enough of the mongrel in him to be a true highway patrolman.

More often than not he would issue cautions rather than fines. He assumed that most drivers were good, honest and hardworking people going about their day and did not see the need to crucify them for minor indiscretions on the road. He would first let an offending driver undertake the attitude test. This occurred within the first ten seconds of meeting, and was not always undertaken by verbal responses. Often it was assessed by body language. If a driver said 'You're just picking on me,' or 'Why don't you get a real job?' or 'Fuck me mate, I wasn't doing anything wrong. Give me a break,' then Rowdy would mentally stamp their licence with 'fail'. Rowdy would then issue the driver with as many infringement notices as possible. On the other side of the coin, if a driver were to throw their hands into the air in defeat and reply with, 'You got me. Sorry mate, I was a bit quick there,' then they would have a very good chance of receiving a caution. If Rowdy came across that same person a second time, however, they would not be so fortunate.

His method of enforcement was always directed towards improving road safety. If he came across a driver with a smooth tyre then he would always give them the opportunity to change it with the spare before issuing a fine. If Rowdy could get the vehicle roadworthy there and then, he had done more for road safety than issuing a fine and allowing a driver to continue on their journey with a smooth tyre. He would much rather see a person put the money towards a new tyre than a fine.

Rowdy shaved and showered, but his mind was still consumed with the images and sounds of that fatal night and its aftermath. He no longer heard the laughter of his children. He did not reply when they asked him something, leaving them confused. Why did he snap at them or berate them for a minor indiscretion? He did not have the answers and hated himself for the person he was becoming. All his eyes were seeing was death and carnage. Even the day after the pursuit he was required to attend the morgue and identify the body of the deceased. When he arrived the three cavity post mortem was under way. The stomach and chest cavity had been opened to reveal all internal organs. The top of the head had been cut away to expose the brain and the skin of the face peeled forward. When asked to identify the body, all Rowdy could reply was 'Yep, that's him. I'd recognise that foot anywhere.' The body lying before him was unrecognisable except for a severed left foot.

'Have something to eat before you go,' said Emma as she placed some toast on the table.

Rowdy pulled up a chair. 'Just a quick piece or I'll be running late.'

Rowdy picked up his knife to spread the margarine. He paused a moment, starring at the blade. He visualised cutting through his hand to see what it felt like. He knew it would hurt. He knew it would bleed. He knew it would be a stupid thing to do but nonetheless he could not help but imagine doing it.

'Are you alright, love,' Emma again asked, oblivious to what was going on in his mind.

Rowdy kept his inner thoughts to himself. 'Yeah, I'm fine.'

'Don't forget to finish work on time today,' Emma reminded him. 'You're picking the kids up from school and taking them to the dentist for their check-up, remember.'

'I won't forget. I've written myself a note,' replied Rowdy convincingly. He was writing himself notes a lot lately to help him remember things he had to do.

'… and don't forget we have the kids school play tonight at six,' added Emma.

Rowdy's voice was filled with sarcasm when he replied, 'I can't wait.'

6.30AM

Taking in the peaceful surroundings, Ricky stood on his unit's small, back veranda, finishing his bowl of cereal. His unit backed onto paddocks belonging to the Chifley Agricultural Research Station. At the moment the paddocks were filled with grazing sheep.

Further in the distance was the education campus of Chifley College which had started out as the Chifley Teachers College.

The backdrop was the imposing Mount Skyline. The mountain overlooked and kept watch on the town of Chifley like a nurturing mother and its name was boldly emblazoned in white across its slope. It was the annual meeting site for racing enthusiasts, both car and motorcycle, from across the nation. It started in the 1930's when a dirt track was cut into the mountain. The track is now a public road, with a sixty kilometre an hour speed limit, and had numerous private houses, winery and orchards around it.

Twice a year, however, the mountain came alive with more than one hundred and fifty thousand racing enthusiasts. At Easter, the Motorcycle

Grand Prix is held, but it was in October that the Chifley Classic brought the mountain to life when the blue and red battle colours of Ford and General Motors Holden are unfurled for their high octane duel.

Ricky was posted to Chifley from the Police Academy just one year after the mountain experienced its bloodiest battle – in the form of riots. At first, opposing spectators came to vicious blows over who had the best race car. They then combined their forces against a common enemy, the state Police Force.

He received his introduction to race weekends when he arrived in Chifley a week before the October car race. Additional police were brought in from all around the state.

The mountain itself was policed by the Tactical Response Group who would convey offenders down to the local police station twenty four hours a day for every day of the long race weekend. Ricky thought being rostered on night work for his first race weekend would be a quiet shift. He was wrong; it was the busiest, especially in the charge room.

Adjoined to the charge room was the station's prison cell complex, consisting of a large exercise yard with a steel mesh roof leaving it exposed to the elements. The area is merely a void, enclosed by dull and aged concrete walls with no fixtures or fittings of any kind. However, given its location and use, you could say that it was tastefully decorated – there was not one square centimetre of wall space that was not signed, engraved or doodled upon in various colours. Some were just a name and date to mark the author's little place in history. Others were a detailed lament of a life gone wrong. There were even poetic verses written, praising one's criminal achievements. Then there were the usual crude and vulgar remarks intermingled amongst threats made towards their captors. It was a stunning sight, considering all prisoners entering this area had been thoroughly searched, and any property or objects found upon them seized. The only other object in the exercise yard was a secure grill and drain located in the centre of the eighteen square metre concrete floor. This allowed blood, vomit, or any other excrement, to be hosed away.

Three solid steel-plate doors, with hinged inspection flaps lined the back wall of the exercise yard. They led to three individual cells that measured two metres by three, each fitted with all the mod conveniences required to live a happy captive existence.

A stainless steel toilet nestled in one corner. Next to it was a stainless steel hand basin with the luxury of cold water only. A raised, solid concrete platform doubled as a bed and lounge. If you were lucky enough to get the resort suite then it also came with a thin, vinyl covered foam mattress.

On a race weekend, the entire cell complex was filled to capacity. There was standing room only as offenders were packed in, shoulder to shoulder, most in some degree of intoxication. All Ricky did for a solid eight-hour shift was photograph, fingerprint, charge and bail offenders. Each individual offender was formally charged by writing up the offence indictment in the charge book. Charge and bail forms were then typed as fingerprints and a photograph were taken with the identification brooch placed under the offender's chin. The nights were long and tedious.

There were lighter moments, and at times even comical. Once Ricky opened the steel door to the prisoner exercise yard and called out the next offender's name to be processed.

'Billy Blogs, you're up.'

A voice came from amongst the crowd of prisoners. 'That's me. Stand aside, coming through… get out of my way, dickhead.'

Ricky looked down at a document provided by the arresting police, including the attached Polaroid photo of the offender. He took note of the photo so he knew he was getting the right Billy Blogs. When he looked up, he could see people stirring and moving sideways, but no one appeared to be making their way forward.

Ricky called out. 'Hurry up, Billy. The quicker we start this the sooner you get out.'

'Down here dickhead,' came the voice again.

Ricky felt a tug on his trousers. He moved the document he held to one side and looked down. 'Hurry up, dickhead. You're cutt'n into me drink'n time,' said Billy Blogs as he looked up at Ricky. Sitting, at Ricky's feet was a man with both legs amputated half-way above the knees. Ricky looked back at the Polaroid. He looked back at Billy.

'You've got no legs,' Ricky said in surprise.

'Shit no. I'd like to report a steal'n. Some bastard stole me legs,' Billy said, to the laughter of all the other prisoners.

Ricky's surprised look turned to confusion. 'It says here you were arrested for driving a motor vehicle in a manner dangerous.'

'Jesus, another fuck'n Einstein,' Billy replied over the laughter. 'How'd ya expect me to catch the bastard that stole me legs, run after him.'

Composing himself from his own fit of laughter, Ricky duly charged Billy Blogs, the man with no legs, for doing doughnuts in his modified car amongst tents and campers on Mount Skyline.

Ricky turned his back to Mount Skyline. A broad smile was painted across his face after recalling the man with no legs. With an empty cereal bowl in hand he stepped back inside his unit, washed his dishes and grabbed his car keys.

Dick opened his eyes as the first rays of sunlight filtered through the curtains. The left side of his face was buried deep in his pillow, his body contorted to find a comfortable position on the bed. Through blurry vision, he noticed a small mark appear on the wall, adjacent to his bed. At first he thought it was his eyes playing tricks on him with the pillow half obscuring his vision.

He lifted his head off the pillow and concentrated on the mark with a squint. The mark began to slowly grow in size. It radiated from the centre, like a droplet of ink absorbed by paper. Dick raised his upper body onto his left arm and stretched across the gap between bed and wall. His right hand reached out. He placed the tip of his index finger onto the expanding stain, and then lightly dragged it downwards.

He reached back and rubbed the thick warm moisture between index finger and thumb. It had a smooth slippery texture. He raised his finger hesitantly to his nose and took a shallow inhale. Dick did not detect any particular odour. A deeper, longer smell this time and maybe a hint of rusty iron filled his nostrils. He then placed his finger onto the tip of his tongue and was immediately met with a biting metallic flavour. It was similar to when he was a child and placed his tongue on both positive and negative contacts of a small nine volt battery as a dare from a friend. It did not have the same tang as the battery but there was certainly that same residual after-taste.

He swung his legs over the side of his bed and planted both feet on the soft carpeted floor. He leant forward again to peer more closely at the broadening stain. He noticed the colour was dark brown with a tint of red. It now began to spread more rapidly. It was no longer just a stain; it now oozed and dripped down the wall like a waterfall in slow motion.

'It's blood,' Dick exclaimed as the realisation hit him.

The plaster was now becoming so soaked with blood that it started to crumble to the floor. Dick leapt upright and began tearing away chunks of plaster, exposing the timber frame of the house. He gasped in shock as his eyes fixed on those of another. They were the eyes of death, starring but without seeing. The face they belonged to had the bluish, leaden colour of lividity. Pulling away more plaster revealed a body.

He now pulled away larger and larger chunks of wall. More and more bodies were exposed within the cavity. Some were fully clothed, while others partly, in torn and tattered fabric that may have once resembled garments. Others were naked and in various stages of decay.

Rotting flesh and maggots fell from some, and bones rattled as skeletal remains collapsed as they were uncovered, free from their tomb.

He worked frantically now until every wall in his room was devoid of its lining. His chest heaved as he panted and gulped for air. Sweat streamed down his naked torso as he turned to every wall and took in its macabre scene.

Dick looked down at his wife who slept undisturbed and innocent of his grizzly find. He made a move to wake her, but then stopped himself mid-stride. He realised it would be best to dispose of all the bodies first so as not to frighten and distress her. He decided to go get his wheelbarrow and strode into the hallway that ran through the centre of the house. He noticed multiple stains appearing on its walls. Like the first, they gradually started, then grew faster and faster until joining with the next. He again started his frenzied work to tear off the walls. Again, body after body was revealed. Every room he went into was the same. Even the kitchen cupboards were packed with distorted and folded bodies. Torn limbs filled the draws.

The bedrooms of his seventeen year old daughter and fourteen year old son did not escape Dick's destruction and gruesome finds. He was astounded, but thankful his children were not woken by his labour. His entire house was littered with remains of plaster. Not one wall was left intact. He tore away the last shred of plaster lining. The body it revealed let out a deep, gut wrenching satanic laugh that echoed through the house.

Dick sat bolt upright in bed, as the echoing sounds of his nightmare reverberated through his head. Sweat oozed from every pore of his body, soaking his pyjamas and staining the bed sheets. He panted rapidly for breath as he realised he was in the safety of his bed and the walls, as he looked around the room were intact and unblemished.

Every night had been the same now for more years than Dick could remember. If it was not bodies in his wall cavities, then it would be some other similarly bazaar nightmare to torture his sleep. It was at the stage now that he would avoid going to bed.

He would stay as active as possible until one or two in the morning. He believed that he would be so exhausted he would just sleep and not have to face the horrors of the night. The result was always the same – his mind never turned off during those resting hours, which were consumed with fear, panic and revulsion.

Dick had been a member of the state Police Force for twenty-one years. At forty-two years of age he still only held the rank of senior constable. He had not necessarily been left behind by the promotion system; he chose not to be a part of it. The promotion system had changed several times over his career, which had seen him perform various roles. He was now the Scene of Crime Officer with the Coal Valley Local Area Command stationed at Brookstone.

Lack of ability did not prevent him from being promoted. He was a very dedicated police officer who gave his full commitment to any role he was assigned. He was the type who came to work every day and did his job well, while those around him spent more time looking for the next one. As new bosses came and went, Dick always impressed them with his demeanour. His bearing and manners were beyond reproach, and the hierarchy would often receive complementary remarks from those he came into contact with. His professionalism, courtesy, honesty, and calm persona would often aid individuals in times of stress.

The honesty component of his character was one of his most dominant traits. Through his work as a Scene of Crime Officer, Dick was in a unique position that necessitated access to members of the public's most private possessions, most often their homes. He was required to perform delicate assessments that ensured correct cataloguing of evidence with minimal disturbance and disruption to the victim. Dick did this time and time again, the victim always leaving with a positive attitude towards him and the organisation for whom he worked. He was meticulous and proficient when it came to record keeping, which was vital to his role.

Feeling utterly exhausted, Dick gingerly got up from his bed. He slowly made his way to the bathroom where he was overcome by nausea. He rushed to the toilet bowl and emptied the contents of his stomach in several loud and painful reaches.

Bent over the vanity, Dick rinsed his mouth with water and spat to remove the fowl acid taste from his mouth. He raised his head slowly and said to his reflection in the mirror, 'Only thirteen more years of this shit to go and you can retire early on a full pension. Just get through another day.'

His reflection showed grey flecked heavily through hair not yet starting to thin. His body was still trim and showed no signs of middle age spread, however, it was taking on a frail appearance as muscle definition was starting to wilt. In fact, Dick was actually six kilograms lighter than when he enlisted all those years ago.

Dick's wife appeared in his reflection beside him. A gentle hand gave a loving rub to his back. 'Why don't you take the day off?'

Being the loyal employee that he was, he replied, 'No-one will do the work for me. It'll still be waiting for me when I go back and that only means the victims who have been broken into will have to wait longer. They've already suffered enough.'

'You've been sick a lot lately,' said his wife, full of concern. 'At least go see a doctor.'

'Probably just something I ate, I'll be OK now it's gone.'

Dick had not told his wife about the nightmares he experienced. He did not want to burden and worry her with his problems. In fact, he rarely told his wife any of the things he experienced at work in any great detail. They were too horrific for the average person to deal with. What he did not realise, or chose not to believe, was that he was just an average person, the only difference being the uniform he wore.

'Do you feel up to some breakfast?' his wife asked.

'I'll grab a quick bite after I shave and shower.'

'You've got plenty of time. You don't start till eight; sit and relax while I fix your breakfast.'

'How often do I sit and relax?' he inquired of his wife's reflection.

Her face brightened. 'Well, today can be the day,' she said happily and patted his back as she left for the kitchen.

Dick continued to look at his own reflection, but now with an inquisitive eye. He could not work out if the face he was looking at was older than he felt, or if he felt older than he looked. The one thing he did see in his mirror image was an emotionless shell, reflecting a man whose life had become totally reliant on routine in order to function. But Dick was not functioning, at least not in an emotional sense. His physical side was able to get about the day and give the resemblance of normality but his mind, his analytical and decision making ability, were at breaking point.

'Bring on retirement,' Dick said to himself, wishing away the next thirteen years of his life. He opened the vanity cabinet mounted on the wall and started his daily routine.

Rowdy downed his piece of toast in several bites and did not waste too much time chewing. Washing it down with a gulp of orange juice, he went to the bathroom. He buttoned his starched and pressed police shirt, stopping long enough to take a quick glance in the mirror to check all was in order. He then pulled a T-shirt over his head and straightened it over his police shirt. He would spend the next eight-hour shift standing out in a crowd because of the uniform he wore and the high visibility car he drove. If he could spend the next fifteen minutes driving to work as anonymously as the next person, that was a good start to the day.

'Dentist. School play... got it.' He kissed Emma on the cheek goodbye. Anne and Jordan gave their father a hug and kiss. Rowdy said, 'Be good for mum and don't be late for the school bus.'

The family lived at the small rural village of Marwood, ten kilometres out of Bowen, their nearest town. The school bus picked the kids up at their front gate, taking about an hour to do its rounds before dropping the children off at school in Bowen.

Rowdy left for the twenty kilometre drive into Benstown where he was stationed. As he drove, his mind was occupied with all the outstanding reports, statements, and files that he had to catch up on.

The clock mounted on the kitchen wall in the Mater household neared seven. Its matriarch, Roslyn, was already behind schedule for the day. Normally she was up around five-thirty with her husband Franco. She found that this was the only quiet hour of the day she had to converse with her husband. With four girls under nine and still trying to complete the home they were owner-building, days tended to be hectic from start to finish.

Today, however, she had slept through the alarm that woke Franco so he could prepare for work. She only stirred when she felt the moist warm lips of her husband as he kissed her cheek goodbye. She had missed cooking Franco his hearty breakfast whilst chatting together to catch up on each other's lives as husband and wife, rather than as mum and dad.

The first load of washing would normally be in the machine, and she would have started on three of her children's school lunches with their school bags lined along the kitchen counter.

Roslyn and Franco had purchased twenty acres of land near Bowen some years ago. Their ambition had always been to live on acreage, build their dream home and raise a large family in a safe rural environment.

They wanted to fill their lives with small pleasures like collecting freshly laid eggs or tending to and nurturing a bountiful vegetable garden. The children could care for a menagerie of animals, catch yabbies in the dam and have the freedom to explore the environment that surrounded them.

This fantasy was now becoming a reality. The couple had all but built their dream home. They had put their soul into its construction with copious amounts of sweat and tears lost along the way. Although the house was not completely finished, it was habitable and they moved in only one month ago. Compared to the shed they had been living in for the past two years, it felt like a palace.

Roslyn made her way from bedroom to bedroom, waking her precious girls. Just before stirring each, she would pause and smile at their innocent youth, wondering what new and exciting discoveries they would make today.

Ricky drove towards Chifley Police Station, whistling and singing to the latest number one hit that pulsed from his car speakers. He ran through in his mind what he wanted to achieve at work today. He always set himself goals to attain in his day, however he was flexible enough to realise that he did not always have control over the way his day would pan out. It was one of the things he loved about being a policeman; you did not know what to expect next.

No other traffic was in sight when he pulled up at a red stop light. Comfortable in the anonymity that the confines of his car provided, he continued his singing as he tapped his hands on the steering wheel to the beat of the music.

Another vehicle pulled up in the lane on his right. He glanced over to see the driver looking at him. Feeling somewhat self-conscious, he stopped singing but continued his drumming as he looked back up at the red light. He felt himself still being watched. He again glanced to his side to find the driver still gazing upon him, this time with a sour look. Ricky returned a pleasant smile and gave a brief greeting wave. With a final look laced with arrogance, the other driver did not return the gesture and looked away. He must not like mornings, Ricky thought to himself.

The traffic light turned green. As if on the starting grid of the Chifley Classic, the other car was quick to accelerate, leaving Ricky behind. The accelerating car reached the speed limit, and then had to brake. Ricky watched as the brake lights came on and the nose of the car dipped to stop from exceeding the speed limit. The realisation that he was wearing his police uniform suddenly struck. Even in his car, where most of his body was obscured, the blue-marle shirt that he wore, with the police insignia patch proudly displayed at his shoulder, could be clearly seen over the window sill and attracted people's attention like steel to a magnet.

Ricky laughed out loud. He could hear the words spoken to him by his Chief Inspector on his first day at Chifley, as they walked together in full regalia through the main street. 'Son,' the Chief Inspector said, '… if it feels like everyone is looking at you, then that's because they are.' He was never to forget these words of advice for his entire career.

Ricky drove past the impressive and imposing Chifley Court House. The grandeur of the structure never ceased to captivate him, particularly when it was him climbing its steps to enter through the domed foyer into the courtroom to give evidence. He could visualise those police from another era who had done the same. He was proud to walk in their ghostly footsteps and be part of the history of this old building. Completed in 1880, in Victorian Renaissance style, the Courthouse was one of the best examples of nineteenth century public building architecture in the state.

Ricky was actually impressed with Chifley as a whole. Having only heard of the city prior to his police posting there, he knew nothing of the history of this large country town.

Discovered in 1815 on the banks of a meandering river, Chifley boomed during the gold rush days of the 1850's and 60's. Unlike many of its surrounding hamlets that declined as gold ran dry, Chifley still prospered today as one of Australia's fastest growing modern regional cities supported by cattle, sheep, wheat, vegetables, and fruit farming.

'I'm on a good thing here,' he murmured as he drove through the synchronised blend of old and new around him.

Ricky parked his car at the front of the old Chifley Police Station. As he locked his door behind him, the town echoed with the toll of bells from the nearby carillon, striking its hourly tune.

7AM

Rowdy walked through the back door of Benstown Police Station into what used to be an old laundry. The station was far from being a purpose built, modern and efficient state-of-the-art complex. Had it not been for the illuminated police sign out the front, anyone passing would have taken it for another old home on suburban Hunter Street. In fact, that's just what it was.

Back in the days when Benstown was a growing rural community, the local policeman, or Lock-up Keeper as he was known, lived in the residence with his family. Attached to the home was a small lock-up where he could perform his constabulary role with sufficient room for detaining prisoners, drunks, and vagrants. The constable's wife would then be responsible for feeding any person detained in custody.

The old residence, still with its original cedar doors and panelling, had undergone numerous refurbishments, extensions, and renovations over the years as the town and its contingent of police grew. Today it houses, in a rabbit warren of disjointed rooms, a Chief Inspector, three administration staff, a Station Sergeant, eleven General Duty police, five Highway Patrol officers, three Detectives, an Intelligence Officer, and the Police Prosecutor on court days. Add to that a locker room, charge room, exhibit rooms, secure firearm loading facility, public counter area, and waiting room, along with a fleet of police vehicles and modern electronic equipment that is essential to life in the modern world. The old residence had long outlived its intended purpose. It is even remarkable that the building is still standing, given its termite infestation.

Benstown is a boom town. From its beginnings in the 1820's the area provided some of the best grazing land in the Coal Valley region. Although the town is still well regarded for its beef and cattle industry, it is mining and power generation that are the town's two largest employment providers. The military also plays an important economic role in the town's existence with a training centre and live bombing range located on its outskirts.

Rowdy strode past the meal room. The familiar and jovial voice of Sergeant Dunnell Wilkins greeted him as he flashed past the door.

'Morning, Rowdy.' Rowdy stopped and back tracked several paces to peer into the kitchen where he saw his Station Sergeant perusing the local paper as he sipped his morning coffee.

'Morning, sarge,' Rowdy replied as he walked into the meal room. 'Anything of interest in the paper?'

'Nothing that we don't already know about,' the sergeant replied.

'Takes the fun out of reading the paper when we supply half the news for them.' He took a seat opposite and placed his well-used sports bag on the floor beside the chair.

Sergeant Wilkins tilted his head down and peered over the top of his reading glasses. 'There's a small article here about you and that little incident of yours,' he said referring to Rowdy's fatal pursuit. 'You even appeared on the morning's national news coverage.'

'Yeah, I caught a glimpse,' replied Rowdy. He did not need to see the media coverage to relive that fateful night.

'It's good that everything turned out okay in the end.'

'I suppose so,' replied Rowdy vacantly.

The old sergeant had known Rowdy for years. As with all the junior troops, he was always concerned about his welfare. He had seen first hand what Rowdy had to endure over the last eight months since the fatal pursuit.

He had witnessed the stress and trauma caused, not just by the pursuit and how it ended, but by the subsequent investigation and the inquest. Decisions that were made in split seconds at the time were later scrutinised, analysed, and brought into question with the benefit of time and in the safety of a sterile courtroom. He knew that police and men in general did not seek or ask for help readily. They would battle on in silence whilst experiencing inner turmoil.

Sergeant Wilkins removed his glasses and looked directly at Rowdy, seeing through his façade. 'Don't beat yourself up over it, Rowdy,' he said with a shake of his balding head. 'You've been around long enough to know that we can't really control any of these incidents we go to. All we do is respond to what someone else is doing, particularly with pursuits. We are powerless to stop them. All we can do is follow them until that person decides to stop, or crashes.'

Rowdy's hands opened and closed several times into tight fists as he sat with his arms outstretched across the table. 'I know, I know. I've been telling myself that for eight months.'

Sergeant Wilkins continued his advice. '… and if they do crash, we can only pray they don't injure or kill some innocent person. Be thankful that in your case it was the offender who was killed and not some innocent bastard.' To an outsider listening to this conversation, the advice may sound callous, but Rowdy knew from a police perspective it was the only way you could look at it.

'Thanks,sarge,' Rowdy replied, managing a smile. 'Thanks for the motivational pep talk first thing in the morning.'

Sergeant Wilkins placed his glasses back on his nose, adjusted them into place and looked back at his newspaper. 'Well I've got to talk to some bastard. There's no-one else here.' He turned a page.

'Where's the GD crew?'

'They don't start until ten,' Sergeant Wilkins replied, a touch of annoyance was obvious.

Rowdy was to jinx himself when he replied, 'What, doesn't anything happen before ten?'

'Apparently not, according to the stats the intel computer spits out,' Sergeant Wilkins pushed his chair back to get up.

'God help us all,' said Rowdy. He rose out of his chair, grabbing his sports bag on the way up.

Sergeant Wilkins poured his cold coffee into the sink. 'God help *me* you mean,' he said, rinsing his cup. 'I've got to supervise you for the next three hours until some real police start work. I've just finished reading about the trouble you highway blokes cause.'

Rowdy headed towards the door and stopped in its opening. 'You'll be happy to know then, that I've been tasked on a seatbelt enforcement today. What possible trouble could I cause doing that?'

Sergeant Wilkins yelled as Rowdy disappeared out through the door, 'Just remember, I'm watching you.'

Rowdy had a lot of time for the old Sergeant and held him in high regard. When outside of work he would call him by his first name, or 'Dunny', as was common amongst his friends. But when at work, he would always respect the rank that he held and addressed him accordingly. Importantly, Rowdy respected the man.

Ricky ran across the road from his parked car and into the driveway of Chifley Police Station. He had no particular reason to race across the road as there was no traffic to beat at this time of the morning. He had the energy and enthusiasm provided by his youthful years to burn and enjoy, and he was keen to start work.

He entered the rear compound of the station and slowed to a brisk walk as he passed the demountable building that housed the detectives. Chifley Station was like many older stations that were once a residence and left behind by the growth of a town. The modified police station was now too small to comfortably accommodate its contingent of police. The old troopers' horse paddock at the rear had long been covered by concrete and built upon while the old lock-up had experienced several refits. He entered the change room and found that his offsider for the day was already dressed and ready for work.

'Morning, Tombstone,' Ricky said cheerfully.

Tombstone was a senior constable with nearly twenty years in the job. He was due for promotion to sergeant at any time.

'Ricky,' came Tombstone's greeting in a deep voice that was never wasted on the use of too many words and even less syllables. 'You're with me.'

His cheerful expression remained spread across his face. Ricky replied with a hint of sarcasm, 'Great.' He actually enjoyed working with Tombstone and all his gruffness. He possessed a wealth of knowledge that Ricky tried to siphon. He appreciated his quiet company as it was close to his own reserved nature. He inserted his key and opened his locker. Tombstone left the change room in the direction of the front counter area.

Ricky lifted out his appointment belt from inside his locker. At Chifley, it was customary to hang it from the door by placing the large buckle clips in one of the pressed metal ventilation slits located near the top of the door. The belt was about eight centimetres wide and made from thick heavy leather which, if properly cared for, would last an officer's entire career. Attached to the belt was a hardened leather gun holster which housed his thirty-eight Smith & Wesson, fully loaded, six shot revolver.

It was widely joked that you could do more damage to an offender by throwing the revolver at them. Not known for its stopping power, however, the revolver was reliable and more importantly, *copper* proof. Fitted to the front of the belt was a small leather pouch which carried a speed loading strip with a further six rounds for the revolver.

On the opposite side to the holster was the handcuff pouch, along with two ring clips secured by leather straps. One was used to carry a torch while the other was for sliding in a rolled aluminium long baton. These two items were not personal issue but carried in all police vehicles and able to be grabbed upon exiting. The trousers Ricky wore were old stock. They had the old rubber baton sleeve sewn into the leg so the truncheon could be carried out of sight.

Ricky eagerly placed the gun belt around his waist, oblivious to its weight. He secured the buckle at the front and then placed four press studded leather keepers around the belt which secured it to his inner belt that was threaded through his trousers.

He picked up his hard-peaked antron cap, with its blue and white checked band, closed the locker door and headed off in the same direction as Tombstone.

Ricky entered the main station area where Tombstone and the officer rostered for station duty for the shift were standing either side of the Station Sergeant at the front counter. They were examining a book of some kind, flicking through the pages.

'Get the ruler and red pen, Ricky,' the Station Sergeant said on hearing Ricky enter.

'What's up?' Ricky enquired.

'We have an important ceremony to perform.' He handed him pen and ruler. 'We just received an all stations telex message. A copper at Redfern had a heart attack and died.'

Ricky was at first shocked, not by the news itself but at how lightly the sergeant referred to it. 'That's terrible news, how old was he?'

The sergeant grinned, his expression turning serious when he answered Ricky, 'Don't worry about his age son. It's his rank that's important.'

Ricky was confused. 'What's his rank got to do with him being dead?'

'The stud book, Ricky... the stud book,' Tombstone said with rare excitement. He assumed it must be important for Tombstone to show this much interest.

The stud book listed the name and registered number of every member of the force. As promotion was based on years of service, if someone died who was senior to you then that put you up one notch higher in the stud book and closer to promotion.

The sergeant placed the ruler across the page and drew a bold red line through the dead officer's name and details. In a solemn tone he then said, 'May he rest in peace,' and lowered his head in respect.

'May he rest in peace,' recited both Tombstone and the Station Officer with their heads bowed.

'Was he senior to me?' Ricky asked with enthusiasm after a suitable period of mourning that lasted for several seconds, had passed.

The three officers standing before him raised their bowed heads, looked at Ricky and then burst into laughter.

'Son, everyone is senior to you,' said the Station Sergeant.

'Yeah, even the police dog is senior to you, Ricky,' quipped the Station Officer.

Ricky was keen and ambitious to work his way up the ranks. He had not given much thought, however, to whether he wanted to be the capstone of the Police Force. But, like they say, if you are going to think, you may as well think big. 'So I'm one step closer to being the Commissioner of Police?' he enquired.

'That's right son,' replied the sergeant.

'I like that ceremony then,' said Ricky with a smile. The fate of the dead officer was already a distant memory.

'It's alright for some,' mumbled Tombstone with remorse. 'The bastard was junior to me.'

The room again erupted into laughter, drowning out the telephone that rang at the main switch, lost amongst the wisecracks darting from one officer to the other. The telephone continued to ring and the Station Officer, whose job it was to answer incoming calls and take care of counter enquires from the public, made no attempt to answer it.

'Are you going to get that or should I?' Ricky asked.

'What possible good could come from answering the phone.' Ricky had noticed that it was a common trend amongst the older police to avoid answering the telephone. At times he had seen those police leave the front counter area if a member of the public was seen approaching the front door. He did not understand why. Ricky had often heard police talk about stress and how the job wears you down. Stress was just a foreign concept to Ricky though, and he did not believe in it. He formed the opinion that these police were just lazy, and vowed he would never become like them.

As the three senior officers continued to exchange light hearted banter, Ricky answered the telephone. After a short conversation and some scribbled note taking, Ricky disconnected the call. He turned to Tombstone and said, 'We've got a cot death.'

The laughter stopped as abruptly as it had started. The three senior police instantly transformed into the professionals that they were. 'Just leave your notes, Ricky. I'll type up the telephone message pad,' said the

Station Officer and fed a piece of paper into the typewriter sitting on the front counter.

Every phone call that came into the station had to be recorded and actioned. Tombstone and Ricky were the only General Duties police working today and the job would be allocated to them. 'Grab the keys, Ricky, you're driving,' Tombstone said as he placed a report of death form in his clip folder.

As Tombstone and Ricky left for their police vehicle parked at the rear of the station, the voice of the Station Officer could be heard following them as it echoed down the passageway, 'I told you no good would come from answering.'

Rowdy stood in front of his locker on which one of his talented and artistic colleagues had practised their graffiti artwork. Emblazoned across the top of the locker was his nickname. It was written in a loud flamboyant style, accentuated boldly by every coloured highlight marker its creator could lay their hands upon.

If you were not aware of that fine Aussie slang tradition of allocating a nickname to someone based on substitution, comparison or irony, then you would easily think Rowdy was the life of the party. In fact he was the complete opposite. Early on in his career, Rowdy was christened with his nickname because of his quiet and reserved nature. He was always conservative and restrained in his behaviour and the fact that he did not drink alcohol only added to his rowdy reputation.

He could not help but chuckle as he looked around at the names on the other lockers. You had the traditional 'Bluey' for the red-headed fiery bloke. 'Phantom' was Bryan's nickname because you could never find him. 'Johno', another of his Highway Patrol offsiders, had the double nickname of 'Bootlace' because he was always tied up every time you asked him to do something. There was 'Toad', 'Frog' and 'Benson' who's reasoning for their creation had been long lost to history.

Rowdy removed the T-shirt from over his police shirt and placed it in his locker, grabbed his gun belt and buckled it around his slim waist.

'I remember when I couldn't wait to get this thing on,' he said to the empty room. 'Now I can't wait to get the bloody thing off.' He wriggled it around to try and relieve the twinge he felt in his hips. He walked to the adjoining gun room where he unlocked the large steel safe that secured all firearms. With another key, he unlocked the padlock securing his gun to its holding peg and removed the Glock 22 semi-automatic pistol. He placed the muzzle of the pistol into the steel cylinder of the safe loading dock, which was surrounded by sandbags and had a wad of telephone books inserted in it to absorb any bullet that may have been accidentally discharged.

Without having to think, Rowdy automatically went through the loading procedure and racked the slide of the pistol three times, locking it open after the third. Checking the pistol was not loaded, he heard himself shouting in his head the drill, 'Look Check. Feel Check. Clear.'

Satisfied the pistol was free of any rounds and obstructions, Rowdy inserted a full fifteen shot magazine of forty calibre rounds inside the hand grip. He then released the slide forward, chambering a round, and pulled it back slightly to check that a round was correctly bedded in. Now fully loaded and operational, Rowdy removed the muzzle of the pistol from the loading dock and holstered it. He quickly checked the additional fifteen round magazine that he carried on his belt, removed his capsicum spray canister and shook it to mix its contents before use.

Next on the checklist were his handcuffs and he ensured the steel bracelets were unlocked and the ratchet mechanism worked correctly and smoothly. He returned them to their double pouch, which also contained his personal protective equipment.

Satisfied that everything was in its place and operating correctly, Rowdy left the room five kilograms heavier and headed to the Highway Patrol office.

7.30AM

Roslyn Mater had just finished hanging out her first load of washing and returned to the kitchen. Her three school aged daughters sat at the breakfast table in the large, eat-in kitchen, giggling excitedly amongst themselves as they ate their cereal.

'You three are in a good mood this morning.'

'I was just practising the poem that I have to say in class today,' replied eight-year old Sophie.

'Must be a funny one for your sisters to be giggling,' said Roslyn, packing a school bag.

Sophie crossed her arms and pouted her lips sulkily. 'It's not supposed to be, mummy, but Sarah and Jenny kept making funny faces at me while I was saying it.'

Roslyn stopped what she was doing and turned on the children with a serious look. 'Is that right, you two?'

Sarah who was six and Jenny five both stopped their giggling and with contrite expression crossing their faces looked down in unison. 'Yes, mummy.'

'Well that's good then,' Roslyn said brightly. 'Your sister needs a distracting audience to practice in front of.'

Realising they were not in trouble, the girls faces beamed again. They lifted their heads and continued to pull faces at their older sister.

'You're acting like children again,' Sophie said in a mature voice. Her composure did not last long as she quickly joined in the laughter.

'Who's for toast then?' Roslyn asked.

'I am...' 'Me...' 'Yes please,' came a trio of replies.

Roslyn placed four slices of bread into the toaster.

'Will you be a big help to mummy, Jenny, and get the Vegemite out of the fridge?'

Her face beamed at having been singled out to assist, over her older siblings. She leapt from her chair and ran to the fridge. The door swung open, followed by a swoosh of cold air. Little Jenny stumbled backwards, still holding the door handle, and regained her balance. Then, standing on tip toes, she stretched to her full height, just managing to grasp the jar , and ran back to the breakfast table.

Roslyn said, 'You forgot to close the fridge door.'

Jenny raced back, slammed the door closed and returned to her seat as her mother was placing the toast on the table. 'I'm mummy's little helper,' Jenny said proudly, with a nod of her head towards her sisters.

'You're all mummy's helpers,' Roslyn said with encouragement. 'Now finish your breakfast and then get dressed for school.'

Roslyn went to her youngest daughter's bedroom where two-year old Teagan was still soundly sleeping in her Barbie doll bed. Roslyn had been up numerous times during the night to sooth her crying. She diagnosed that her daughter was suffering an ear infection, probably picked up from all the swimming they had been doing lately. Roslyn had given her an infant pain reliever after which she had settled into an undisturbed sleep. With no reason to wake her, Roslyn returned to the kitchen.

All three girls had the spread smeared from the corners of their mouth. Jenny had eaten the centre out of her toast and was making shapes out of the crust as she twisted it in her hands. 'Wipe your faces, teeth and when you're dressed, we'll get your hair done,' said Roslyn to prompt them to their rooms.

'Okay, mummy,' replied Sophie and climbed off her chair. Her two younger sisters followed her lead and raced each other down the hallway, giggling all the way.

Roslyn stood in the empty kitchen and with some relief murmured, 'I should check the street number. I must be in the wrong house. No fights or arguments this morning.'

The washing machine beeped to signal it had finished another load. Any thoughts that she was in the wrong house soon vanished.

Dick drove north on the Great North Highway through Benstown as he made his way to Brookstone, another forty kilometres away. He was the sole Scene of Crime Officer commonly reduced to SOC officer for the Coal Valley Local Area Command or LAC. His role included attendance at crime scenes to gather any fingerprint or DNA evidence left behind by an offender. He made detailed written notes and photographed the scene and any evidence, for later production at court.

He enjoyed the role, working well alone, and with a LAC covering thousands of square kilometres, there was plenty of time to be alone just in travel time. An average day could see Dick travel to all extremities of the command area.

As SOC officer, he was part of the Crime Management Unit of the command. His function was to support the general duties police, detectives, and highway patrol officers in their day-to-day investigations. Whether it be a break and enter, stolen car, armed hold up, home invasion, or drug related crime, Dick would be there, providing his expertise. Even after an offender was arrested, he was involved in performing the forensic procedure to obtain that person's DNA for comparison with that found at a crime scene.

It was a role he was quite happy to perform for the remaining years of his service but this was another aspect of his life he was unable to control. The latest trend of the Police Service was to civilianise the SOC officer role. Rather than have police perform this function, it was cheaper to employ university graduates, usually with a background in the sciences who were not only paid less, there was no initial training and ongoing costs associated with being a police officer. The Coal Valley LAC was one of the few commands not to have its police SOC officer replaced with a civilian. The prospect of returning to general duties policing horrified him. These days, Dick avoided confrontational situations. He found he could no longer attend the likes of domestic disputes and follow due process as he once could.

Dick had never been a physical or violent person, but his internal thoughts increasingly wanted him to be. He would now have to tell himself not to do something, or react in a certain way, when once it was not even a passing thought. Returning to general duties was not an option for Dick. As he drove to work, he ran through what options he still had but he kept coming up with the same answer – none.

'You should have got on the promotion elevator, my boy,' he said to himself as he stopped at a red light.

A young couple stopped their car beside his. Dick looked across and saw them engaged in jovial conversation and laughter, revelling in each other's company, oblivious to the outside world. He wondered how long has it been since he felt like that?

It had been that long he could not remember. He was unable to recall even what that feeling of euphoria was like. He was just floating through life on autopilot. He had built this protective wall around himself for so long now that he felt nothing. He could not even see over his wall, let alone climb and escape.

'Your first cot death?' Tombstone asked.

'Yeah, I've heard of Sudden Infant Death Syndrome but have never experienced it,' replied Ricky. Like most recruits prior to joining the police force, Ricky had no experience with death from any cause. It was just something he saw on the television news.

'You're not alone there,' Tombstone continued. 'It's a mystery to the top doctors and scientists worldwide.'

'Don't they know what causes it?' asked Ricky.

'No, not really. Death is sudden and usually in otherwise healthy babies,' said Tombstone. '…makes it one of the greatest misfortunes that a family can suffer.'

'So the baby has no symptoms before it happens?' enquired Ricky, keen to learn from Tombstone's knowledge and experience.

'No warning signs whatsoever, and as far as I know it is impossible to predict. Don't think it's restricted to babies either. It can strike anytime up to about two years of age,' said Tombstone.

With three children of his own he had lived in fear of SIDS, but all his children had passed through the danger period.

'So how do we know it's a SIDS death or not?'

Tombstone smiled, pleased his young offsider was thinking.

'Initially we don't. We have to investigate the scene, carefully interview the parents, and obtain a medical history of the child. We wait for the autopsy results and if the doctors can't establish a cause of death, then SIDS is given as the cause,' said Tombstone.

Ricky hesitated before commenting, 'It really is a mystery then?'

The two officers continued their journey in comfortable silence. Ricky knew Tombstone was a lot like himself. Not a great conversationalist when in mixed company, but one on one he was more than willing to converse on a more personal level.

'You seem to handle this death thing pretty well. What's your secret?' Ricky asked.

'No secret, son. It's just something you have to deal with in your own way,' Tombstone replied with a shrug of his shoulders.

'Do they affect you?' Ricky persisted.

'Every one of them affects me. I might not show it, but I care about people you know. That's where a lot of coppers, I think, make a mistake. It's better to feel emotion than to not feel it at all. It makes you better at your job.'

'But you can't get emotionally involved in every job you do, can you?' Ricky delved deeper for an answer.

'Don't confuse feeling emotion with a personal attachment to a job. The two are completely separate. You still have to create a barrier around yourself that detaches you from your work. You don't allow it to attach to the point where you take it home. If you do, you'll end up like Billy Dorsman,' replied Tombstone.

'Is that Senior Constable Dorsman whose name appears on the roster every day?' asked Ricky with interest.

'Yep,' replied Tombstone.

'I've been here over twelve months and I've never laid eyes on him,' Ricky said.

'He's on long term sick report,' explained Tombstone.

'What made him sick?' enquired Ricky.

'The job,' Tombstone replied, and then added, 'Stress. Mad as a cut snake.'

Ricky continued to probe into Tombstone's mind. 'You don't believe in stress do you?'

Tombstone did not hesitate in his reply. 'I do. What's important though, is how you deal with it.' Aware of Ricky's gaze, he added sternly, '…and watch the road. Stick around long enough, son, and you'll understand one day.'

The two men again travelled in silence.

'I've solved two mysteries today already,' said Ricky as he turned into Bentinck Street.

Tombstone sighed before reluctantly asking, 'What are they?'

'The first is the mystery of Billy Dorsman.'

Ricky waited for Tombstone to ask what the second mystery was, but Tombstone remained quiet as he looked for house numbers. When he could not wait any longer, he said, 'Don't you want to know what the second is?'

'Not really, but I'm sure you're going to tell me.' By this time, Tombstone could not wait to get out of the police truck and do the cot death, just to escape the questioning. He had shared more of his thoughts in the last few minutes than he had done in the previous twelve months.

'I've discovered that you're capable of talking in sentences.'

It was Tombstone's turn to give Ricky a critical look. 'You know Ricky, you can be a real little prick that gets under the skin.'

Tombstone looked towards the row of houses and pointed to number fifty-four.

Roslyn finished plaiting Jenny's long blonde hair. She glanced up at the wall clock. 'Time to go kids,' she yelled towards the lounge room, where Sophie and Sarah were watching television after having had their own hair brushed and braided. Normally, Roslyn would walk all four children down their four-hundred metre gravel driveway to the front gateway to catch the school bus into Bowen. It was nearly eight o'clock though, and the bus usually arrived a few minutes after.

'Go hop in the car girls. We'll miss the bus if we walk today,' said Roslyn over her shoulder as she walked to Teagan's room to check on her sleeping daughter.

She found Teagan still fast asleep. Roslyn left her undisturbed.

'Good girls. You've got your seat belts on already,' Roslyn said after she opened the tailgate of her four-wheel-drive and threw three backpacks in. Roslyn jumped up into the driver's seat and started the vehicle. As she accelerated down the driveway, Roslyn pushed the button that wound down her driver's door window and let the cool fresh morning air fill the cabin.

'Mummy, you haven't got your seat belt on,' said Sophie from her seat in the back and with the wind blowing on her face.

'Mummy will be okay until we get to the gate honey,' replied Roslyn as she continued to accelerate along the meandering driveway.

Roslyn's mind was occupied with thoughts of her kids missing the school bus and Teagan waking up to find no one in the house. She pushed the accelerator harder.

8AM

Roslyn approached a right-hand bend in the driveway as the front gateway came into sight from between the trees and shrubs that filled the front of the property.

She realised she was going too fast for the bend and jabbed at the brake pedal. It was too late. The large, heavy vehicle had already entered the bend. The instant she applied the brakes, the rear tyres lost traction on the loose gravel. The back of the car swung violently to the left. The three girls sitting shoulder to shoulder across the back seat screamed.

Roslyn frantically turned the steering wheel to the left to correct the sliding vehicle. The left rear wheel ploughed sideways into the stony dish drain that ran the length of the driveway. The rear of the four-wheel-drive then whipped suddenly to the right.

The steering wheel could not be turned quickly enough the other way to steer into the slide. The rear of the vehicle swung until it was finally travelling broadside down the gravel. The vehicle was lost in a cloud of dust as pebbles hurtled from under tyres that threatened to peel from their rims.

Large boulders were in place along the dish drain every twenty metres to slow down the flow of water during heavy rain. The four-wheel-drive whipped to the left again. A front tyre struck a boulder as the car again entered the drain. The effect was devastating. The bottom half of the vehicle slowed but the high centre of gravity continued its forward momentum.

The four-wheel-drive rolled sideways as it was thrown into the air. The girls screamed now in terror as their bodies were forced against the seat belts. The school backpacks were tossed about the rear cargo area. The steel mesh cargo barrier, fitted behind the rear seats, dented under the force of the bags but held firm.

Roslyn tried to turn around to see her children, but everything was just a blur and her lungs filled with dust. She was totally disorientated as the vehicle toppled. Her hands gripped the steering wheel until her fingers turned white. Her foot continued to press harder onto the brake pedal, unaware the wheels were no longer on the ground.

The large vehicle continued to roll sideways. Roslyn's unrestrained body was lifted out of her seat. Her head and shoulders started to pass through the open window. The driver's side of the vehicle then struck the ground. Roslyn was killed instantly as her head was crushed between the top of the door frame and the ground. The sides of her head distorted as her skull smashed into fragments.

The crumpled vehicle completed a full roll. Over two tonne in weight, the four-wheel-drive settled back heavily onto its wheels that sagged with broken suspension. The vehicle rocked, absorbing the last of its momentum in a cloud of dust.

The three girls were thrown to one side for the last time and all became quiet and still. They were covered in diamonds of glass from the windows that had exploded under the collapsing roof of the vehicle as it somersaulted. Apart from a few bruises caused by knocking into each other, Sophie, Sarah and Jenny were alive. They were all shaking uncontrollably as they sobbed, unable to scream any more.

Sophie looked into the front of the vehicle through teary eyes and the mist of dust that filled the cabin. She saw her mother slumped forward. Roslyn's hands were still clutching the steering wheel in a death grip while her head rested on the steering wheel between her arms.

Her long black hair covered her face and hid the horrific injuries. 'Are you alright, mummy?' Sophie asked hesitantly.

There was no reply. Sophie unbuckled her seat belt. With her younger siblings still sobbing, Sophie leant through the gap between the two front seats.

'Wake up mummy,' she said as she reached through and shook her mother's shoulder.

Only silence greeted her again.

'Mummy, wake up!' Sophie said more forcefully and pulled back on her mother's shoulder.

Sophie pulled with such adrenaline fuelled force that she pulled her mother off the steering wheel. Roslyn's lifeless body flopped against the back rest of the driver's seat. Her distorted skull struck the head rest and fell forward again.

Sophie saw the left side of her mother's bloodied face.

'Aaaah!' She could only gasp as she reeled back from the shocking sight. Her reaction to scream was voiceless. She starred in utter confusion that numbed her body.

The piercing squeal of brakes and the sharp sound of escaping air penetrated Sophie's trance as the Bowen school bus pulled to a stop at the front gateway.

Sophie quickly swung into action and unbuckled her younger sister's seat belts. She grabbed Sarah's hand, kicked open the side door, and pulled her sister out of the vehicle behind her. Sophie reached back into the four-wheel-drive as Jenny climbed across the seat towards her. Grabbing her little sister, Sophie carried her while holding Sarah's hand and started to run down the driveway towards the bus.

Sharon had been driving the Bowen school bus for ten years and knew every one of her young passengers by name. As she approached the Mater's gateway she noticed that the three eldest girls were not sitting on the timber fence rail, swinging their legs as they did most mornings. Roslyn was normally standing nearby, nursing young Teagan. If it had been raining, Teagan would be jumping in muddy puddles.

Sharon stopped the bus level with the gateway, and looked up the gravel driveway. She noticed the white four-wheel-drive parked at an odd angle, just off to the side about fifty metres from the entranceway. A gentle breeze was blowing a cloud of dust away from the vehicle. She saw no-one nearby. Then, concentrating her vision onto the vehicle, she noticed its roof was damaged and collapsed at all four corners.

A hiss of air escaped as Sharon pushed a button on the console and the concertina automatic door opposite opened with a jerk. She stepped down from her seat and stood in the open doorway. Confused, she watched as Sophie stumbled from a rear door of the vehicle with her sister Sarah in tow.

'Everyone stay in your seats and on the bus,' Sharon calmly told her half full bus of primary school children. She stepped down onto the roadside with one hand still holding onto a grab rail mounted inside the bus. The full realisation of what had happened then struck her.

'Oh my God, no,' Sharon yelled as she started running towards the four-wheel-drive. All the children on the bus rushed to one side and lined their faces against the glass to see what was happening. Two of the faces that peered through the hand-smudged glass belonged to Anne and Jordan. Rowdy's two children had been picked up by Sharon only minutes before.

'Mummy won't wake up,' Sophie said to Sharon in a shaking voice as they met.

Sharon noticed that Jenny, who had her arms firmly wrapped around Sophie's neck and shoulders, had a lump on her forehead the size of a golf ball. Sarah, who was still holding her big sisters hand, had small cuts and scratches on her face. Sharon then saw the children's school uniforms sparkling, as tiny shards of glass reflected the sun.

Forcing herself to remain calm and not let the fear swelling inside paint her face, Sharon told Sophie, 'Take your sisters to the bus. I'll check on your mum.'

Sharon approached the driver's door of the dented vehicle. She could see a figure with its head bowed. Fearing the worst, she covered the last ten metres running. The image that greeted her, when she stopped and placed her hands on the driver's door window sill, was worse than any she could imagine. Her first reaction was to look away from the grizzly sight. Even though her appearance suggested otherwise, Sharon was compelled to check if Roslyn was still alive.

Swallowing deeply the bile that rose in her throat, Sharon slowly reached up and brushed aside Roslyn's hair with a shaking hand. She searched for a pulse in Roslyn's neck. The skin was warm and supple. There was no pulse. Sharon ran back to the school bus and used its two-way radio to call for help.

After parking his car, Dick walked to the rear entrance of Brookstone Police Station. He entered his security code into the electronic door lock. The locking mechanism immediately disengaged and he pushed the door inwards. Dressed in shorts, T-shirt and thongs, Dick looked like any other person who had been walking along the street. He was fit and healthy for forty-two and carried no excess weight. When he walked, however, it was with a slightly discernible limp from hip pain, which always felt worse than it visibly appeared.

With a battered sports bag in hand, he headed to the change room inside the newly purpose built double storey police complex. The ultra-modern building had been built on the same site as the old Brookstone lock-up. With the old building heritage listed, most of its outer façade could not be demolished but the architects had blended the old with the new, highlighting the old. The glass and steel structure that dominated the site grew from the back of the old brick station as easily and pleasing to the eye as a new limb shoots from the stem of a tree. The ground floor housed the local Brookstone Police Station while the first floor was the command centre for the entire Coal Valley Local Area Command, which controlled eleven police stations in all.

Dick placed his sports bag onto a table inside the change room and unlocked his locker door, where everything inside had a place, neat and tidy. Unzipping his bag, he rummaged through it and removed his dark blue police overalls, placing them on the table. He removed his T-shirt, then his shorts – it was always in that order. Dick often thought about being adventurous by removing his shorts before his T-shirt, but never did. Who knows what would happen if he did? The earth may stop rotating and it would be his entire fault.

Dick had the misguided belief that this routine and daily ritual was one of the few things that he could actually control in his day. Once he walked out into that station, who knows what he would be doing or where he would be going.

The reality was that there was still something controlling him. He was not even free to choose how he undressed. His mind and body were being manipulated by a force that he could not see, touch, hear, or smell.

After having suited up and finished tying the laces on his GP boots, Dick walked to his office and sat down in front of the computer. He entered his password and registered number into the system. He browsed through the list of events that had occurred over the length and breadth of the command in the last twenty-four hours.

'It's been a quiet night,' Dick said to his empty office.

Dick only had one job to attend which was a break and enter locally in Brookstone. The rest of the events listed were the usual – offensive behaviour, noise complaints, assault police, and drink driving charges – none of which required his expertise.

It was going to be the perfect day to play catch-up. Dick had numerous requests from police to provide a statement for court on crime scenes that he had examined. He had a fridge full of DNA samples requiring individual Exhibit Examination Forms prepared and sent on to the analytical laboratory in Sydney for analysis and profiling.

Dick smiled as he swivelled his chair away from the computer, relishing the thought of a quiet day in the office. He stood from his chair and considered what to do first. 'It must be time for a cup of coffee,' he murmured.

Rowdy sat in his highway patrol office typing furiously at thirty-five words a minute. He had decided to finish a brief of evidence, which was due for submission, prior to hitting the road on the seat belt enforcement he was rostered for.

Like all police, Rowdy had a backlog of paperwork. Every day he had all the good intentions of catching up. No matter how hard he tried, though, he just never caught up. The end result of most days was he had more paperwork to do than at the start.

Today was going to be different. He was the only highway patrol officer in the office, at least for the next few hours anyway, until Bryan and Baz were rostered to start.

Rowdy was determined to make the most of his peaceful surroundings and get as much paperwork done as possible. He was confident the motoring public of Benstown would not miss his presence on the road, particularly, those not wearing seat belts.

'Benstown 16, or the vehicle covering Bowen, for a motor vehicle accident,' came the radio operator's voice through the ceiling-mounted speaker in his office. Rowdy was deep in concentration as he transferred the words flowing through his mind onto the keyboard as he typed. He was vaguely aware of a mumbled sound in the room.

The radio operator, with no response, again said impassively, 'Benstown 16, or the vehicle covering Bowen, for a fatal accident.'

Rowdy stopped typing this time when he heard the call sign Benstown 16. He sat staring at the blinking cursor on his computer screen as the reality of his earlier conversation with Sergeant Wilkins registered. There was no Benstown 16 starting until ten and no vehicle was working Bowen today, both its officers had the day off. The intel computer said nothing happens today until after ten am.

Rowdy looked up from his computer as the imposing figure of Sergeant Wilkins filled the doorway. 'Looks like we've got a job, Rowdy,' said the Station Sergeant.

'Righto,' Rowdy said with some frustration. He clicked *save* on the computer. 'So much for that then.'

'We'll take your car if that's okay?' asked the sergeant.

'Fine… I'm ready to go whenever you are.' Rowdy stood and took the car keys off the keyboard mounted on a wall.

'I'll get my gun on and then I'm right to go,' said Sergeant Wilkins patting his hips as if to check what was there. The sergeant's role did not require him to leave the office that often. He saw no reason to lug around an extra five kilos about his waist. He was yet to find a use for his service pistol indoors, except maybe as a paper weight.

'Meet you out the back,' Rowdy said as he grabbed his work bag. He followed Wilkins as he headed back towards his own office. 'Sarge, you do know where your gun is, don't you?'

Sergeant Wilkins stopped and looked towards the ceiling, as if in thought before replying. 'I think so. I'm pretty sure I took it out of the kid's toy box last year and put it into the safe.' He changed directions and headed towards the gun safe room.

Rowdy walked into the main station area and picked up the police radio handpiece from its cradle. 'Benstown 202 radio, leaving Benstown Station. Two up.'

After briefly speaking with the parents and ambulance officers who were leaving, Ricky and Tombstone stood just inside the bedroom door. Their eyes darted around the small bedroom. They first looked from side-to-side, then, from floor-to-ceiling.

'Nothing looks out of the ordinary,' Tombstone said flatly.

'Apart from the dead'n in the middle of the room,' said Ricky as he pointed towards the blue, lifeless infant that lay in a cot. Most occupations tend to develop a language all of their own. The police force was no different with its unique jargon. *Dead'n* was one of those common terms used, and was in no way said in a derogatory manner.

'I can see that,' Tombstone said as he turned to look down the hallway towards the sobbing parents to check they were still out of ear shot. 'We're looking for something else, remember. Anything that doesn't fit, or out of place. Don't forget why we're here.'

Ricky felt angry with himself that he had to be reminded of his job. He had let his feelings of compassion and sorrow for a devastated family blind him. His role was to investigate a death, not simply take a report of it. There was always a chance that something more sinister has taken place here. 'You're right... sorry Tombstone.'

He realised he still had a long way to go in this job and a lot to learn. It was the seasoned professionals like Tombstone who were not about to let him forget, either.

'Dust off that notebook of yours,' Tombstone said sharply. 'Record everything. Draw a diagram of the room if you have to.'

Ricky now treated the room as a crime scene and began to make his detailed notes. He approached the cot. The child, who had just turned six months old, lay on his back with his little arms stretched out above his head. He wore a short sleeved jumpsuit with a coloured cartoon character embroidered on it. His eyes were closed. Had it not been for the bluish discolouration of the skin and lips, he looked to be sleeping peacefully.

The side of the cot was down. The light-weight bed sheet and blanket were made up from the bottom half of the cot only and were turned down to expose the child's body.

When they had arrived at the house, the mother had told Ricky that she breastfed her son about five, changed his nappy and firmly tucked him back into bed. She went back to bed only to be woken around six forty-five by the shouts of her husband to call an ambulance. When she went to her son's room she saw her husband giving mouth to mouth to their son. The ambulance arrived within minutes of the phone call, but could do nothing to revive the child, who was already dead.

'Are you ready to do the identification statement?' asked Tombstone. A formal identification of the body was required to be given to police. The police officer to whom the deceased was identified, was then required to identify the body to the forensic pathologist in order for an autopsy to be performed.

'Yeah,' replied Ricky without enthusiasm.

'I'll bring the parents in,' said Tombstone. 'After the ID is done, let them hold their child if they want to. It'll be the last chance they get before the body snatchers arrive.' Tombstone always referred to the local funeral directors in this way.

'I still have to get a statement from the parents about what happened,' said Ricky.

'I'll get the father's version. You get mum's,' Tombstone said, giving Ricky the harder of the two statements to obtain.

If getting someone to identify their dead six-months old son was not bad enough, Ricky knew that dealing with the grieving mother was going to be difficult. He could already feel the shame swell within him, knowing the questions he would have to ask her.

The trauma she would be put through would only be compounded when she had this young, twenty-one year old police officer trying to give words of comfort and support. Ricky could not even begin to imagine how this young couple must be feeling. The protective wall that was starting to be built around Ricky, just had another layer added as he prepared himself for the unpleasant task ahead.

'Don't forget to obtain a detailed medical history on the boy. Infections, accidents, medications, anything,' instructed Tombstone as he left the bedroom and walked down the hallway towards the grief stricken parents.

8.30AM

Dick walked back to his office with a steaming coffee mug firmly grasped in his hand. He quickly passed the doorway leading into the front counter area of Brookstone Police Station when he heard the uproar of cheers, laughter, and applause. Back-peddling, Dick stood in the opening to see one of the General Duty police taking a bow like a jester in a medieval court.

'Well done, Billy,' shouted one officer as he applauded.

'Onya, Billy,' cheered another over the laughter.

At the centre of attention was Billy Lang. Billy was a senior constable with twenty five years' service and had just doubled back onto day work after knocking off at half past eleven the previous night. Unfortunately for Billy, the news had already spread rapidly about one of his jobs he'd attended last night.

'Hey Dick,' one of the GD's called after spotting him in the doorway. 'Come and hear what Billy the Pervert got up to last night.'

'Don't you mean, who he got up,' roared another.

Dick usually avoided the front station area of any police station these days but intrigued by the jovial atmosphere, he entered. He did not have to answer the phone, take counter enquiries or respond to that section of the community who found it impossible to run their lives without involving the police in some way. As he mingled with the uniformed GD's and took a sip from his mug, one of the gathering said, 'Go on, Billy. Tell us all what happened last night.'

'Get comfortable Dick,' another GD said. 'You know what Storm Cloud Billy is like when he gets an audience.' Billy was the type who was always moaning about things. Every work place has one. It was said that if you got at the right angle and the light was right, you could actually see the storm cloud hovering above his head. It followed him everywhere he went, drizzling rain onto his balding crown. Bolts of lightning flashed in all directions above him and thunder rumbled on with each step he took. To top it off, Billy just happened to be a Pom – a whinging Pom, with a starched British accent.

'Now, now gentlemen,' said Billy aloofly as he prepared to recount the events his colleagues found so entertaining. The gathered crowd of six quietened, Billy cleared his throat and began.

'It all started around three when I had the unfortunate experience of being rostered to work with that new female probationary constable. Well I can only assume she's female as she was wearing culottes, but to look at her you...'

'Christ, Billy, get to the good bit. We all have to knock off sometime today,' one said, cutting Billy off.

'If you insist,' Billy continued in his aristocratic tone. 'At nine-oh-one my colleague and I received a call from radio about a disturbance in the public amenities building located in the park. The radio operator was vague on details, so we attended with undue haste and on the way...'

Billy was again cut short when an officer quipped, 'If you don't get to the toilet block in undue haste, Billy, there'll be a disturbance right here.'

'Very well,' said Billy as he raised his hands in front of his chest in a calming motion. 'As I approached the building, with the stealth of a tiger stalking its prey, I heard a sickening groan come from within. I immediately thought the worst. It was obvious some hideous crime had taken place, leaving some person in dire need of urgent medical assistance. Without a thought to my own safety or well-being, I raced to his aid with cheetah-like speed. My visually displeasing colleague would later describe me as a blur on the face of the wind. I covered the last two metres to the entrance with the theme song from Chariots of Fire spurring me on.'

'Does this show come with an intermission,' Dick interjected with a sour look, after taking a sip from his mug. 'My coffee has gone cold.'

Billy looked at him with a grin and said, 'Patience my dear man. The climax is near.'

'Upon entering the brightly lit confines of the privy,' continued Billy, 'my vision was momentarily obscured. Instinctively, my hand firmly encircled the moulded grip of my service pistol as I shielded my eyes from the fluorescent glare with the other. As my twenty-twenty sight returned, I was confronted with two startled male faces, which at first glance appeared attached to the same body. The faces and body were motionless, like a kangaroo mesmerised by headlights. Then, as the entirety of the scene developed, I observed that it was in fact two bodies in close proximity to each other like conjoined twins at the waist. I then observed a disturbing fact. Surrounding the ankles of each set of hairy legs, lay the crumpled trousers and undergarments of their owners, who stood, front to back, in shocked euphoria. 'Hello, hello, what's going on here then,' I yelled.'

'Lucky you didn't yell, *Fuck me*, Billy or you would have been in real strife,' one of the GD's laughed.

Billy continued as the uproar around him subsided. 'There was only one thing that any self-respecting officer of the Crown could do in the circumstances. I made a tactical withdrawal and ran away faster than I entered.'

The gathering again burst into uncontrolled laughter, bringing some to tears. Dick placed his coffee mug on the table he rested on then straightened and walked over to Billy. Placing one hand on Billy's shoulder and shaking his hand vigorously with the other, Dick said in a serious tone, 'Billy, I'll type the report today. There'll be a Command Citation in this for you. You've gone where no other police officer in this command has dared to go. You might even get a medal if I leave the bit out about running away.'

Dick could not believe that no-one in the last six months, since Billy had transferred to Brookstone, had told him about that toilet block. He retrieved his mug and turned to leave the jovial crowd when one of the older men approached him.

'Before you go Dick, take this survey form,' said the officer. He took the document from him.

'What is it?'

'The department's Healthy Lifestyle rep was here yesterday. He was interested to know if any police here had been involved in any traumatic events,' replied the GD with a bewildered look and shake of the head.

'Jesus,' Dick replied with a chuckle. 'A roll of toilet paper wouldn't be long enough to list the traumatic events we've been to.'

'Yeah, and that's only in the last twelve months,' the officer added.

Dick looked at the document and read its title. 'Coping with Trauma,' he read aloud. 'Should be interesting,' he continued sarcastically.

He thumbed through the pages which listed forty-two symptoms and reactions to traumatic events. Dick ticked the boxes off in his head as he went through the numerous emotional, physical, behavioural, inner thoughts, and dreams categories listed on the form.

'What happens if you tick them all?'

'Then you're fucked…. just like the rest of us,' the GD officer said with an understanding smile.

'That's comforting to know,' Dick replied as he filed the survey into the garbage bin. He may not have been so dismissive of the document if he had read the paragraph that mentioned if you suffered from two or more of the listed symptoms over a period lasting longer than five to six weeks, then you were at risk of suffering severe depression or anxiety. It recommended that you should seek professional assistance. In Dick's case, most of the symptoms had been with him for years.

Sporadic laughter still drifted from the station area. He mumbled under his breath to the demons that controlled his life, 'I'm not going to let you bastards beat me.'

'Benstown 202, off at McCauley Road, Bowen,' Rowdy informed the radio operator as he parked his highway patrol car near the wreckage of Roslyn's four-wheel-drive.

An ambulance was already on scene with a small girl being treated in the back for cuts and abrasions to her head. The local fire brigade were also on scene. The brigade captain greeted Sergeant Wilkins and Rowdy.

'What have we got?' Sergeant Wilkins asked after shaking hands.

'One female driver deceased and still in the vehicle. Three of her daughters have cuts and bruises but otherwise okay. There is also a two year old girl up at the house. I have one of my boys up there with her.'

'Why is the school bus here?' Rowdy asked as he looked down the driveway towards the bus he had driven around to enter the property.

'The driver called the accident in. She stayed with the kids until the ambo arrived,' explained the Fire Captain.

Rowdy continued to look towards the school bus, moving his head forward as if to get a better look. He saw a row of faces and hands pressed against the windows. His eye's widened as he recognised two smiling faces with hands frantically waving towards him.

'Oh my God… no!' Rowdy exclaimed as he recognised Anne and Jordan. 'Did the kids in the bus see the accident,' Rowdy quickly turned and asked the Fire Captain.

'No. The driver kept them on the bus and the kids can't see into the car from this angle,' the captain answered and indicated the direction with his arm.

'Where's Sharon, the bus driver?' Rowdy fired another question as an empty school bus arrived and parked behind the other.

'She's sitting in the ambulance. She's still shaking,' the Fire Captain explained. 'The other two kids are in the front with her.'

'Back in a tick, sarge,' Rowdy said over his shoulder. He started to jog down the driveway.

Rowdy stepped into the bus. 'Can I turn the lights and sirens on daddy?' Jordan yelled excitedly as he ran down the centre isle of the bus to his father.

'Sorry son, not today,' Rowdy replied with a smile as he crouched down to be at eye level with his son.

'Is everybody alright dad?' Anne asked as she walked up behind her brother.

'Yes honey, everyone is fine,' Rowdy lied. To Rowdy's relief it was obvious by all the noise that the kids thought the whole situation was all very exciting.

'I'll see the both of you after school when I pick you up and will explain everything then,' he said as he stood up and gave both a hug.

Rowdy could already imagine the adventure stories that all the kids would have to tell when they got to school. The innocence of youth was a wonderful thing, he thought. It protected them from the harsh realities of life and death, at least for now.

The relief bus driver then stepped up into the bus. Rather than have all the kids change buses, the relief driver told Rowdy he would drive Sharon's bus and continue the bus route to school.

Rowdy stood in the driveway entrance as the bus noisily accelerated away. He returned the waves from excited children as each window passed.

'Wouldn't it be great to be a kid again,' he said out loud to himself as he watched the young ones jostle for position across the back seat of the bus to get one more wave in. 'Not a care in the world.'

'The husband of the deceased has been contacted and will be here shortly,' Sergeant Wilkins explained to Rowdy on his return. 'I'm about to take a statement from the bus driver. The three girls have been taken up to the house. I'll wait till dad or some other relative arrives before I speak with them.'

'How far away are the crashies?' Rowdy asked.

The Crash Investigation Unit was based about an hour away in Kingstown. The police attached to this section had specialised training and knowledge in the investigation of motor vehicle collisions and would normally take over the investigation into fatal accidents.

'They're not interested,' replied Sergeant Wilkins with a shake of his head. 'Because this happened on private property and the only vehicle involved is that of the deceased, there's no criminal liability to investigate.'

'It's a pity we can't take a pass on the job too,' Rowdy said with a hint of seriousness in his voice.

'Crime Scene from Valesville is coming, though. They're only about five minutes away. At least they will take the photos and do all the measurements for the coroner's brief,' said Sergeant Wilkins.

Valesville was the next major town between Bowen and Kingstown. Just like Kingstown it had a permanent crime scene unit stationed there, staffed by three officers.

'The Fire Captain said one of his boys knows the dead'n,' Sergeant Wilkins added.

'I'll get an ID statement from him while you speak with Sharon,' said Rowdy.

'It'll save adding to the husband's trauma. We don't want the last image etched into his memory of his wife to be this one,' Rowdy added as he looked over at Roslyn's horrific head injuries.

This was a decision Rowdy made, not just in the best interest of the dead woman's husband, but also his own. It was going to be much easier for Rowdy to take an ID statement from one of the firies than deal with the emotions of a distraught husband.

'Good idea,' responded Sergeant Wilkins without hesitation. He then started to chuckle. 'That old saying about a wife on her wedding day is pretty true.'

Rowdy was slow to catch on and had to ask, 'What saying is that?'

'You know the one,' the old sergeant said and tossed his head in the direction of Roslyn's bloodied head. 'About how the best your wife ever looks is on her wedding day. It's all downhill from then on.'

'You're a sick man, Sarge… a very sick man.'

Rowdy knew Sergeant Wilkins did not mean what he said. Humour was just one of those coping skills that all emergency service personnel use when confronted with the most horrific scenes. Rowdy started to walk in the direction of the Fire Captain.

'One last thing Rowdy,' said Sergeant Wilkins, causing Rowdy to stop and turn around. 'Get them to put a tarp over her when you're done.'

Rowdy gestured a thumbs up. 'Will do.'

One of the fire officers had known Roslyn and the family for five years. His own children went to little athletics with the Maters and would often be at each other's homes for barbecues.

Rowdy walked the fire officer over to the driver's door of the crumpled four wheel drive and went through the identification process.

As he wrote the last word of the ID statement in his notebook and placed the full stop, the fire officer quickly ran to some nearby bushes. Bent over with a hand on each knee, the officer began to bring up the contents of his stomach.

After the fourth heave, he spat several times to remove the last remnants from his mouth. He slowly straightened, breathing deeply as tears caused by the exertion streamed from his eyes.

Rowdy, still standing next to the driver's door, looked across at the nauseated fire officer. He returned his gaze to the distorted and crumpled vision of Roslyn. Rowdy suddenly felt unsettled. The image that he saw would be forever engraved into his mind. Whether his eyes were open or closed, he could not undo what he had seen. It was not what he was looking at that caused his uneasiness. It was what he was feeling – he felt nothing. He was not shocked or repulsed by the sight. He did not see a loving mother and wife. All he saw was a job to be done and procedures to be followed. The thought of four young girls growing towards womanhood without the help, advice, and support of a caring mother did not fill him with sorrow or empathy. There was no disbelief at what had happened. Rowdy just accepted that these things do happen. Already he had seen it countless times before.

Rowdy was consumed with a coldness that was slowly consuming all aspects of his life. The only things that lurked deep inside the emotionless pit within him were shame and anger. The shame he felt for being so helpless in these situations and the anger towards himself for being the heartless person he was becoming.

Ricky and Tombstone finished obtaining statements from the parents of the dead infant. They stood silently together in the living room of the home, waiting patiently while the parents held and said their goodbyes to their only child. A knock at the front door broke the uncomfortable silence. 'That should be the body snatchers,' whispered Tombstone and moved towards the door.

Standing on the other side of the door were two neatly groomed men. One was short in stature while the other would have to duck when entering. Their facial features were gaunt and sullen. Both could have benefited from going up a size in their suits which did nothing to hide their skeletal frames.

'Good morning gentlemen,' Tombstone greeted as he opened the door.

The shorter employee of the local funeral director offered a bony hand to shake.

'Sorry for the delay.' The deep voice surprised Tombstone, given his diminutive size. 'We've been flat out.'

'I'm pleased to see business is booming,' replied Tombstone dryly.

Tombstone stepped aside and ushered the two men inside. They entered with a rattle as they manoeuvred the gurney they pushed, over the threshold.

Tombstone gave Ricky a nod of his head in the direction of the bedroom. Without a word exchanged, Ricky walked down the hallway and entered the bedroom. The mother was cradling her son in her arms. On seeing Ricky enter, she delicately placed her dead child back into the cot and tucked him into the bed sheets. She kissed his forehead before straightening, and then looked at Ricky blankly.

'If you're ready,' said Ricky softly. 'The funeral directors are here.'

The mother collapsed into her husband's arms, her face buried into his chest, muffling the sobs that shook her body.

The couple walked slowly from the room, clutching each other tightly. Ricky had to wipe away his own tears as he imagined how empty their lives must be right now.

Their whole world had collapsed around them, taking a small part of Ricky with it.

Tombstone and the two funeral home employees entered the room.

'Don't forget to grab the sheets and blankets,' said Tombstone.

Because this was an apparent cot death, the procedure was to send all clothing and bedding along with the body to Glebe Morgue in Sydney for examination. Scientists were still searching for that breakthrough to help prevent this type of death.

In Ricky's short time in the police force he had to touch and handle many dead people. He had even had to search for and pick up various body parts. It never failed to leave him with a dirty feeling. He felt contaminated and could not wait to wash his clothes and take a shower.

Ricky looked on the bright side, though. At least the post mortem would be carried out in Sydney and not locally. If it was performed in Chifley, he would have to attend and identify the body to the doctor performing the autopsy. Although Chifley Base Hospital was a large regional medical facility, it was not overly funded with morgue attendants. In most cases, after completing the body ID, the doctor would get police as his assistant. This required weighing and measuring internal organs as they were removed. Ricky had to take an even longer shower after that.

9AM

The bedside alarm clock increased in pitch as its staccato beep stirred the slumber of Lindsay and Lynda Crisp.

Today was a rare sleep-in for the couple. At this time of year they were normally up at dawn, taking advantage of the cooler mornings to tend to their livestock and market garden. For the hardworking farmers, working with the variety of elements unique to each season was a necessity of life. Today, however, there was to be no hard work.

The couple's only child, twenty-two year old Mark, had spent the last twelve months travelling in Europe. Having completed his agricultural studies, and before he was required to be tied down to the running of the farm, his parents encouraged him to see the world.

His extended working holiday was over, though. Today he was due to fly back into Sydney.

An arm slowly extended from under the bed sheet. A hand groped with searching fingers. The fingers located the source of the noise and in their blind attempt to find the off button, sent the alarm clock tumbling from the bedside table. It was silenced when it struck the floor.

Lindsay's head emerged from under the sheet. He lifted his face off the damp patch on his pillow where saliva had dribbled from the corner of his mouth. His eyes resisted all attempts to open as he squinted against the sun-filled room. His upper body rose onto his elbows, followed by a mouth-widening yawn. One hand rose to massage his unruly hair as his mouth opened and closed in quick succession, trying to regain some moisture to his tongue and lips. He mumbled out loud to himself, 'This sleeping-in caper makes you feel like garbage.'

Lindsay was still groggy from sleep. He turned his head in surprise when his wife lying next to him excitedly said, 'What sleep, I was too excited to sleep.'

Lynda was wide awake and without a hint of fatigue. 'Our little boy will be home today.'

'About time too,' said Lindsay while ruffling his hair again. 'He's been living the playboy life long enough. It's time he did some real work.'

Lynda knew that her husband was just as excited to have their son coming home as she was. He had tossed and turned beside her most of the night trying to get to sleep. It was not until the last few hours that he had fallen soundly off. Not wanting to disturb him, Lynda lay motionless, staring at the ceiling, with visions of greeting her son as he appeared in the arrivals lounge of Sydney Airport dancing through her thoughts.

Rowdy placed a numbered crime scene marker on the gravel driveway where the clearly defined skid marks of the out of control four-wheel-drive first started. He was assisting the Crime Scene officer identify any marks of significance along the driveway in preparation for them to be photographed and measured. The Crime Scene officer would later use his drafting skills to prepare a scaled drawing that would be presented at the Coronial Inquest into Roslyn's death. The drawing would give the magistrate hearing the matter an overall view of the scene in reference to the photographs. The measurements taken would also assist in determining an approximate speed at which the vehicle was travelling when it rolled.

The Crime Scene officer pulled a compass from his pocket and located north. Repositioning the camera slung from his neck, he added to his pages of notes.

'Rowdy,' shouted the Crime Scene officer. 'Remove the tarp from the car, please.'

'Will do,' he replied.

Rowdy had just taken hold of the tarp when his attention was drawn to the roar of a car engine in the distance. Leaving the tarp in place to cover the grizzly scene beneath, Rowdy looked down at the driveway entrance as a car braked heavily, slowing just enough to maintain control as it turned off the bitumen. The engine roared again as the driver accelerated onto the gravel, fishtailing wildly as it stormed across the stony surface. It travelled further sideways than it did forward as the rear wheels struggled for traction. If sound was anything to go by, the car should have been doing one-hundred kilometres an hour. But in the driver's blind haste, he was doing no more than twenty.

'Stop him!' Rowdy yelled to the Fire Captain who was closer to the entrance.

His first concern was to preserve the scene. The last thing he needed was this car driving over all the crime scene markers and destroying vital evidence.

Stopped, the male driver got out of the vehicle and started arguing with the Fire Captain. The man's hands and arms were flailing about at the same pace as his mouth. Rowdy started jogging towards them.

'I need to see my wife!. Where are my kids?' the man yelled.

Rowdy knew that Roslyn's husband had been contacted at his work and was told of the tragic accident. 'Franco, is it?' he calmly asked as he approached.

Franco barrelled past the Fire Captain and walked aggressively towards Rowdy. Both anger and despair showed in his face as he pleaded, 'I want to see my wife!'

Rowdy raised both his hands in front of him in that universal sign to stop and back off. It was obvious, though, that Franco had no intentions of stopping.

'This is my property! I own this land! You can't stop me!' Franco said with determined passion.

Rowdy decided to take the official line. Still with his hands raised and stepping from side to side to match Franco's attempts to walk around him he said, 'Sorry Franco, but I can stop you. This is a crime scene and no-one can enter.'

Franco became enraged. 'What do you mean, crime scene?' he said as he now stood toe to toe with Rowdy. 'No crime has been committed here. My wife is dead! I need to see her.'

Realising he had taken the wrong approach, Rowdy quickly reassessed his options. He could let Franco pass, but in doing so, leave him with the harrowing memory of his wife's crumpled body that the flies were already swarming around, crawling into open wounds.

In order to stop Franco, it was apparent that some level of physical force may be required. If Franco continued to resist, then this physical confrontation would only escalate. The last thing Rowdy wanted was to be wrestling around on the ground at the scene of a tragic accident with a distraught husband.

In the split second it took Rowdy to reassess the situation, his decision was made at the moment Franco again moved to walk around him. He grabbed Franco by each shoulder and faced him, their noses barely inches apart, relieved to feel no real determination on Franco's part to continue as the forward pressure from his body weakened against Rowdy's hands.

'Listen to me, Franco,' Rowdy said, now just resting his hands on Franco's shoulders. 'What you need to do right now is be with your kids. They're scared and they need their father. Let us do our job here. There will be plenty of time later to see your wife. Think of your kids, Franco.'

Rowdy had seen the miracles performed at funeral parlours after bodies had been prepared for family viewings prior to burial. He was confident that Franco would get to say that goodbye to his wife in more fetching appearance and certainly in more dignified surroundings.

Franco briefly dropped his face. When he raised it again, all anger had melted from it. His eyes swelled with tears as he looked back at Rowdy and softly asked, 'Where are the kids?'

Rowdy smiled with relief. 'They're safe, up at the house. We'll get you up there to them.'

Rowdy gently led Franco back towards his car and organised with the Fire Captain to have one of his men drive Franco to the house.

Sergeant Wilkins was already there after having obtained a statement from the bus driver. Sharon had now left in the relief bus. Rowdy was more than confident that Sergeant Wilkins would explain to Franco the legal procedures that would occur. Even though it was obvious how his wife died, the Coroners Act still required the matter to be investigated and an autopsy performed.

'Better him than me,' he said to himself as he walked back towards the four-wheel-drive.

Ricky and Tombstone walked back towards their police truck. Ricky carried a brown paper evidence bag under one arm. It contained the dead child's bed linen along with a small hand knitted fireman doll he had removed from the cot. What had been a gift from a loving grandmother was now part of the investigation into the child's death. Ricky found the doll tucked between the cot mattress and sheets. The parents had calmed down after seeing their son unceremoniously placed into a plastic body bag and taken away. Their emotions again surfaced when they watched Ricky place the doll into the bag, as if all memory of their child was being removed.

The two officers climbed into their vehicle with Ricky placing the evidence bag in the centre of the long bench seat between them. He lifted the radio handpiece and pressed the transmit button. 'Chifley 10 back on,' he said.

Before Ricky could turn the key and start the engine, the voice of the Chifley Station Officer replied, 'Chifley 10. Have a request from Chifley detectives to meet them at the Shell Service Station. You'll be given further information at that location.'

'Chifley 10 copy,' replied Ricky, shooting Tombstone a puzzled look.

Seeing the confused look on Ricky's face, Tombstone helped his young partner out. 'They obviously have something to tell us that they don't want broadcast over the air. Crooks do listen in on scanners you know.'

Ricky was just about to open his mouth and ask Tombstone the obvious question when he glanced across and caught the hostile look Tombstone was giving him. He followed with an equally intimidating comment. 'Don't ask. Just drive.'

Dick had left the relative safety of Brookstone Police Station to drive to his one and only fingerprint job for the day. He was experiencing a rare moment of happiness. The prospect of a quiet day seemed to lift his mood. His spirits were raised further when he turned into what was known locally as the Wine Estate. It was a redeveloped residential area, and the large houses that dotted the estate mostly belonged to people who were generally at the higher end of the social and economic scale. To him, that meant they worked for a living.

There was nothing he enjoyed more than attending a break and enter that had happened to *nice* people who lived in a *nice* home. Even the narrative about the crime that he had read on the computer system was promising. The point of entry to the home was by forcing a locked sliding window open. There was no better surface than glass to leave a fingerprint on. Glass met all the criteria of smooth, clean and shiny that was needed to hold a good print. As in this case with that optimal surface being the point of entry where considerable force is exerted by the hands, then there was an eighty per-cent chance of developing a good, clear and identifiable fingerprint.

Dick turned into Claret Avenue and searched for number ten. He admired the manicured lawns and well-tended gardens decorated with various ornaments, statues and water features. He would occasionally glance at a descending street number that was proudly displayed on an elaborate letter box as he drove slowly along the street.

Dick stopped outside a house he assumed was number ten as there was no street number to indicate. 'I knew it was too good to be true,' he muttered, his mood slumping along with his shoulders. 'Of all the houses in this street, why break into this one?'

Dick stared at the worst house in the best street. An old rusty car body decorated the front yard. The lawn and garden beds were no longer distinguishable, long overgrown with weeds that threatened to consume the house. Most of the front windows were smashed or cracked and had been boarded up on the inside with timber or black plastic.

Remnants of fly screens drooped from their frames or lay on the ground where they had fallen long ago. Timber fascia boards, with only remnants of paint that had mostly blistered and flaked off, skirted the eaves above the red brick dwelling. Guttering had rusted away, no longer capable of channelling water to the outlet where a downpipe was once attached.

One object caught Dick's eye above all others. The dilapidated appearance of the house indicated it may be home to a lazy welfare recipient, but there, mounted on the roof amongst broken tiles, was its crowning glory – the pay TV satellite dish.

Dick stood at the side of his police vehicle. He held a crime scene examination book in his left hand and in the right, a hard black plastic suitcase which contained his fingerprint equipment.

He tilted his head towards the satellite dish. I work for a living and I cannot afford pay TV, he thought to himself.

He slowly made his way through the jungle of the front yard and climbed three steps onto the front veranda, tastefully decorated with an old three seater floral lounge. Its faded and grubby fabric was torn to reveal its yellow foam infill with large chunks missing. Beside the lounge was a large flower pot. Growing from the soil, which was mulched with cigarette butts, was a grey tortured twig, devoid of any leaf matter. It was obviously one of those hardy, drought tolerant shrubs that required little maintenance.

Dick stood before the front door, mustering the courage to knock. Perhaps there will be no-one home, he wishfully thought. Perhaps I've wrongly accused them of being lazy dole bludgers. They may be an unfortunate disabled person who struggles through life doing their best. Or perhaps a struggling family working three jobs to put food on the table and does not have time or resources to maintain the home.

Boosted by these thoughts, Dick placed the crime scene examination book under his right arm. With his left hand now free he gave a loud and confident rap on the door, certain in his belief that this person was in fact in need of his help to catch the unlawful creature who had committed this violation against them.

The door flew open and Dick instantly knew he was wrong and should have stuck with his first assumptions.

'What the fuck do you want?' a man snarled. He stood defiantly, one hand raised holding the door open, the other on the door frame opposite, blocking entry. He was dressed in a torn, faded blue singlet that stretched over an ample stomach, the singlet only just managed to tuck in at the back, into a pair of similarly faded and tattered shorts. At least the man was fortunate that his gut would have obscured the view of his cracked and blackened feet, with their yellow, fungal ridden toenails extending like talons.

The man's mouth was curved in a snarl and revealed more gaps than teeth. His face was covered in a patchwork stubble of growth that reminded Dick of a dog with mange.

'Good morning, Sir,' Dick said politely as he raised a hand to his mouth. The suppressed cough quickly threatened to turn into a reflux gag as he felt the acid bile rise in his throat as the putrid draft of air flowing through the open doorway assaulted him.

Involuntarily he back-pedalled to distance himself from the onslaught of pungent air that was heavy with stale body odour and rotting matter. He wiped the beginnings of a tear in a stinging eye as he continued to say, 'You reported a break and enter to our Police Assistance Line.'

'That's right. Some fuck'n thiev'n bastard stole all me X-box games. Fat lot of good you fuck'n pigs do protect'n us,' said the man with spittle flying from his mouth.

He paused, told himself to remain calm then said, 'Sir, I'm with the Police Fingerprint Section. With your permission I'd like to examine the point of entry. A window I believe.'

'Fuck'n fingerprints,' the toothless man snapped. 'You fuck'n blokes couldn't find a fingerprint if it was stapled to ya arse.'

Dick was always up to the challenge to develop a good identifiable fingerprint, no matter what the circumstances. To then have that fingerprint matched to an offender, and be able to go back to the victim with that information was one of the few rewards the job had to offer these days.

Today was not going to be one of those days. Dick was starting to feel that this turkey deserved to be broken into. The offender was probably only retrieving property that had been stolen from him in the first place. The idiot had already interfered with the peace and tranquillity of his day enough and he started to see a way out of the man's abusive dribble.

'I'm sorry you feel that way, sir. I can't force you to allow me to examine your lovely home, so I will say my goodbyes, but please don't hesitate to call if you need our help in the future,' Dick said, hiding his sarcasm, and turned to leave.

He had taken two steps down the veranda, thinking he had made good his escape.

'Well, ya here now, ya may as well take a fuck'n look,' the toothless man growled.

Dick stopped, his shoulders dropping in disappointment. He turned and faced the man. Forcing a smile, he said with a hint of satire, 'Marvellous. Show me the way.'

Dick followed the man through the front door and was led into the gloom of a dimly lit lounge room. Two ceiling lights were on, but their fifteen watt globes only managed to glow enough to prevent Dick from walking into furniture that cluttered the room. The lounge room had only one external window, and that was draped with black plastic.

'That's the fuck'n window the arseholes broke in through,' the toothless man said as he indicated towards the black plastic.

Dick had been holding his breath since entering the house, however, could still feel the foul smell as it attacked his eyes and skin. Desperate for air, Dick exhaled the last traces of air from his lungs. He was then forced to breathe more deeply than he could control and sucked in the thick air that filled the room. He failed to hold back the cough that came when he said, 'Could you open the blind, please.'

Dick was then enlightened to the intricate workings of the black plastic window covering as the toothless man promptly rolled the plastic up from the bottom, crimped it together in the centre between thumb and forefinger and placed a clothes peg on it to hold it in place.

The room brightened. As the floor and objects around him became distinguishable, Dick's first thought was that someone had been a bit heavy handed with the naphthalene flakes. Everything around him was covered in small white flakes. The soiled carpet, lounges, chairs and timber furniture were all sprinkled like a dusting of snow.

Dick was taken back to his childhood and could see his little old grandmother going around the skirting boards and wardrobes with the naphthalene box, sprinkling sparingly its crystallised contents to ward off silver fish and other small critters. This must have taken dozens of boxes, though. Kilogram boxes at that.

'Did I hear ya talk'n to someone, darl'n,' screeched a female voice from the back of the house after a door slammed closed.

'Yeah, the pigs are here,' the man yelled back.

Two pit bull dogs, one white, the other black, ran into the lounge room and started barking and foaming at the mouth on seeing Dick. The white dog made a run at Dick who reacted by lowering his hard cased fingerprint kit to cover his legs. The toothless man lashed out with one leg and kicked the dog in its midriff. Its snarling was replaced with a yelp of pain as it was knocked off its feet and collided into the leg of a table. Regaining its feet, the dog whimpered away to the other end of the room where it busied itself licking its bruised side.

The black dog continued to growl towards Dick. The toothless man made a rush at it. 'Get out, ya fuck'n mongrel,' he yelled, kicking in its direction. This time he only struck air but the dog retreated and sat by the other dog.

'What do the coppers want?' a woman asked as she entered the room, ignoring Dick's presence.

'He's come to look for fingerprints,' said the toothless man as he nodded in Dick's direction.

The source of the naphthalene flakes now became apparent to Dick as he looked at the female. Dick felt his body shudder under his overalls as he realised the flakes that covered the room was skin. Human skin.

The female's exposed limbs and face were covered in dry flaking skin. She obviously suffered from some sort of skin disorder, hopefully not contagious. Standing there she unconsciously rubbed at her arms, picking off larger flakes.

Dick was paralysed. He had tried to resist the necessity to breath. Now he did not want to move or touch anything. He was trapped in the house of horrors. Just when he thought things could not get worse … they did.

At the edge of his peripheral vision, Dick saw one of the dogs move. Fearing it was about to make another run at him he reached for his capsicum spray. Dick was soon relieved as the black dog began to walk around in circles several times, sniffing at the carpet. Dick's relief then turned to disgust as the black dog squatted. A strained but nervous look settled on its face and its body began to tremble. It evacuated its bowels onto the carpet.

Dick looked around the room and studied it in more detail. The walls were full of holes, probably from being punched or kicked in some drunken rage. Those parts of the wall that were intact were spotted with black mould growth. What glass there was left in the window had a frosted appearance from the build-up of dirt and mould.

'Get me out of here,' Dick's mind yelled.

9.30AM

Within minutes of leaving the Shell Service Station in Chifley, Ricky was standing behind two plain clothes detectives in a hallway of a single level unit block. The meeting at the service station had been brief but sufficient to pass on the details of the meticulously planned operation that was to follow.

Earlier in the morning, Detective Constable James had received information from a local informant that a large quantity of cannabis was being stored in the flat of a local drug dealer. When the Detective quizzed his informant about the information, it turned out the informant had been to the flat to make a purchase. The dealer refused to sell him any as later in the day he was travelling to Sydney where he would get double the price. With a case of sour grapes, the informant promptly contacted detectives.

Within an hour, a statement from the informant had been obtained and a search warrant approved by the Chamber Magistrate. Not wanting to alert the drug dealer to their impending arrival by broadcasting his address over the police radio, the detective organised to meet Ricky and Tombstone at the service station to get their assistance in executing the search warrant.

Detective Sergeant Sims held the search warrant in his hand. The experienced officer made a final check of the address typed on the search warrant. The large black number five screwed onto the outside of the door they stood at satisfied him that all was good to go.

Tombstone had taken up a position at the rear of the flat. His job was to apprehend the drug dealer if he decided to make a run for it.

He casually leant against the outer side of a rear brick wall that surrounded the courtyard of the flat. He passed the time by examining his fingers and performed some relevant cosmetic treatment to his fingernails and hands with his pocket knife.

Sims tested to see if the door handle was locked… it was. Without a word said, he nodded to James to open the door with the key.

Ricky took a step back as the detective raised the ten pound sledge hammer. With eyes focused on the centre of the door handle, he moved his body into the blow. The head of the hammer travelled down in an arc, missed the handle and embedded itself into the hollow core door which remained closed and locked.

When *the key* was used to enter at any search warrant, the person wielding the key had his reputation on the line. The goal was to be a one-key man. That is, one blow, one entry. If two blows of the key were required, then you were a two-key man, and so on.

Today was not the day that Detective James could boast to all who would listen that he was a one key man. He wiggled the handle of the key in a plea to the door to loosen its grip.

As the key was raised for a second time, a high pitched hysterical scream came from behind the door. The second blow found its mark. The handle and lock crumpled. The timber door jamb erupted in splinters as the tongue of the lock tore through it. The door sprang open.

Sims was first through the opening. James followed closely behind, while Ricky stood at the threshold. Sims pulled up short his progress into the flat. Not expecting his sergeant to abruptly stop in front of him James stumbled into his back. The young detective was pumped, primed and ready to chase, tackle and apprehend any person found in the flat. All he could do for the moment was struggle to try and stay upright.

Regaining his balance, James stood to the left of the motionless sergeant. Still cautious, Ricky entered the room slowly, to the right of the sergeant. All three looked at this frightened and screaming young woman sitting on a lounge opposite the front door. Her knees were raised up under her chin and tightly pulled into her chest by encircling arms. Her eyes were closed as she continued to shriek at the top of her voice, tears streaming down her cheeks and her entire body shaking uncontrollably with fear. In her mind she was about to be raped, then murdered.

The young woman's fear was overwhelming. A dark stain began to spread across her jeans and continued onto the lounge as she lost control of her bladder.

'We're the police,' blurted Detective Sergeant Sims, not knowing if to approach the girl or not.

The fear that had taken hold of her body also controlled her mind. She now thought to herself, 'My God, the Police are going to rape and murder me!'

Sims quickly perused the clean and tidy flat. There were rows of what appeared to be family photos hanging from the walls. The coffee table had a pile of student exam papers with Chifley High School letterhead boldly printed on them. The papers appeared to be in the process of being marked. Realising he was not standing in a drug dealer's flat, he moved slowly forward towards the screaming woman. He knelt down on one knee calmly saying, 'You're okay. No one is going to hurt you.'

The young woman opened her eyes. The screaming stopped and was replaced with sobbing between short gasps to breath. Her body trembled, still cowering on the lounge.

'Look, here is my identification,' said the sergeant in a soothing tone as he opened his Police Warrant Card and held it towards the woman. 'Over there is a uniformed police officer. No one is going to hurt you.'

The woman's eyes darted to Ricky who stood with a bewildered look on his face. He had not yet come to the conclusion that they were in the wrong flat. The teary eyes returned to Sims, with her sobs becoming less frequent and softer as her breathing began to settle.

'Wha… what are you doing here?' she whimpered, wiping the moisture from her eyes with an open hand.

'We've made a mistake,' the Sergeant said honestly.

Ricky and Detective James left the flat as their Sergeant continued to explain what happened.

'That didn't go well, I take it,' said Ricky to Detective James.

'No,' the young Detective replied with a concerned look. 'No, it didn't. It took me two swings of the key to get in.'

Ricky shook his head in amazement, unsure if the detective was serious or not.

'I'll go get Tombstone,' Ricky said, and left Detective James who was now looking up and down the hallway, deep in thought.

Ricky finished telling Tombstone about the fiasco as the two detectives returned to the street. The general duties officers were casually leaning on the bonnet of their police truck. Tombstone's face was positively beaming when the two detectives approached. 'Is there anything else we can help you with, sarge?' he managed to say through a smug smile. 'Get you a hammer and some nails perhaps?'

'The real estate agent will take care of the repair work and send us the bill,' the sergeant replied sternly.

Detective James stood with the key propped over one shoulder and said without any indication of embarrassment, 'You know, when we first arrived I had a feeling that I had been to the druggie's flat before and it was number ten, at the other end of the hallway.'

The other three officers just looked at him blankly. The silence was broken when Sims said, 'You idiot. You didn't think to say something before we smashed in the door?'

'The informant said flat five,' James replied.

'That's because he can't count to ten, you idiot.' The sergeant's face reddened with anger.

'Come on Ricky, our work is done,' Tombstone interjected as the sergeant started to wave his finger in the face of his junior officer, struggling to find any appropriate words to say.

Rowdy had just finished talking to Roslyn's parents who had arrived at the property a short time after Franco. Although they were upset and numbed by the death of their daughter, they calmly listened to Rowdy as he told them the circumstances. When they drove up to the house, they gave the crash scene a wide berth by driving through the scrubby paddocks that surrounded it. Given the battered condition of Roslyn's four-wheel-drive, their imagination of the scene within it was bad enough. They knew their place was with the living. They would comfort and support their grandchildren in any way they could and give Franco whatever assistance he required.

'I'm done, Rowdy,' said the Crime Scene officer as he walked over.

'I'll check with radio for an ETA on the body snatchers,' replied Rowdy and started to walk towards his police vehicle. He was halfway to it when a white van turned into the driveway. It displayed no signage of any kind on its panels to advertise its purpose. The only noise it made as it stalked towards its quarry was the crunching of rocks beneath its tyres. Two emotionless faces sat inside with a fixed stare that sent a shiver through Rowdy on a thirty degree day. The funeral contractors approached like crows circling their prey.

Rowdy turned away to break free from their gaze and said to the Crime Scene officer, 'Isn't it creepy how they just appear like that.'

'Both the front doors of the car are jammed and can't be opened,' said the Crime Scene officer to Rowdy, ignoring his comment as he contemplated the body removal.

Rowdy paused as he looked at the crumpled four-wheel-drive and considered the same thing. 'Can we pull her out through the open window?' he now asked.

'I don't think so,' replied the Crime Scene officer. 'The way the roof and top of the door have collapsed would make it impossible.'

Rowdy could picture the grizzly task of pulling the dead weight of a body through the window. He was not happy with what he saw.

'You're right,' agreed Rowdy. 'She's been through enough. I'll get the firies to cut the door off.'

Back inside Chifley Police Station, Ricky sat at a desk furiously typing away to complete the necessary paperwork and bookwork for the cot death. He prepared the P79A Report of Death to Coroner in quadruplicate. The Specimen/Exhibit Examination Form in relation to the doll and bedding was prepared in triplicate and would be forwarded on to the Glebe Morgue. He had taken three photocopies of the identification statement and had typed out the statement contained in his notebook of the mother's version of events. Tombstone had supplied him with four copies of the father's version. Ricky collated the paperwork that surrounded him into organised piles, ready to forward off to their various destinations.

On his way back from the search warrant, Ricky had detoured via the Chifley Base Hospital and collected the certificate prepared by a doctor that pronounced the life of the child *extinct*.

Dick, in his rush to leave the house of horrors, cleared the three steps down from the front veranda without laying a foot on any of them. His arthritic hips stabbed him with pain as they remonstrated against his athleticism. Not wanting to appear desperate, he restrained himself from breaking into a run. He settled for a quick, determined walk that managed to hurdle any junk that lay in his direct path, towards his beckoning police vehicle.

Dick did not turn or glance over his shoulder as he heard the toothless man walk onto the veranda behind him and yell, 'Thanks for noth'n, ya useless bastard!'

Without breaking stride or turning around, Dick raised a hand above his head and waved in acknowledgement. His full concentration was focused on getting to his vehicle, and God help anyone who got in his way. Unlocking his vehicle with a keyless remote, Dick flung open the tailgate and threw his fingerprint case inside. Desperately riffling through the assortment of equipment he carried in the cargo area, he located his spray can of foam disinfectant. Applying a liberal amount into the palm of one hand, he rubbed the white foam all over his hands. Just to be sure he had killed all the bugs and bacteria; he squirted another dollop and massaged the cold alcohol based cleansing solution into his hands again until it had fully evaporated.

Dick climbed into the driver's seat and slammed the door closed. He pushed a button on the door trim and the clunking sound of all the doors locking filled him with relief. He tilted his head back onto the head rest, closed his eyes and sighed. He was at last safe in the confines of the vehicle's cabin. His eyes suddenly opened in a startled expression. The events from the house of horrors had begun to replay on the inside of his eyelids.

He now opened the crime scene examination book and turned to a new page. He began to record the details of his brief examination. Under normal circumstances, he would have done this while still inside the premises in order to be as accurate as possible with his notes. On this occasion, however, the urge to get out of the house overwhelmed the need for accuracy. Dick had performed a less than thorough examination. With all the surfaces being so dirty, the likelihood of developing an identifiable print was minimal. He quickly brushed on some black and white powders, then said to the couple, 'Sorry, no prints. Goodbye,' and had made a dash for the door.

After completing his notes, Dick tossed the examination book onto the seat beside him. He reached for the key he had already inserted into the ignition and was just about to turn it when something caught his eye.

There was movement of some kind on his overalls. He bent forward to the left of the steering wheel and peered down at his legs. There it was again, but still couldn't discern what the movement was. Dick squinted even closer until he could make out the weave pattern in the material that covered his legs. Now that his eyes had focused to see something smaller rather than larger, he let out a cry, 'Oh shit! There's no getting away from this hell hole!'

Dick's legs were covered in fleas. He could now see hundreds of the tiny, wingless, jumping insects. 'Jesus Christ!' he blasphemed at the insects as they jumped about in search of blood.

He frantically searched his arms and upper body for any of the blood sucking creatures. He began to scratch at his scalp and at the back of his neck as his body tingled with that itching sensation that comes just from the sight of the little critters.

Dick's mind began to race. 'What do I do?' he asked himself. Unbelievably, his first thought was to go back into the house of horrors and ask for a can of fly spray. He quickly gave himself a mental slap to rid the thought from his mind. He then considered knocking on a neighbour's door. 'Don't be stupid, Dick,' he told himself. 'What if there's no one home, and if there is, they don't want a flea ridden crazed copper in their home screaming for insect spray,' said his mind.

Dick turned the ignition key and the vehicle roared to life. He slammed the gear lever into drive and planted his foot. The fully marked, police four-wheel-drive lunged forward. Its tyres squealed, leaving a trail of rubber in their wake.

Dick pulled out into the traffic lane and activated his emergency lights and sirens. After all, this was a matter of life and death. Dick could see the coroner's report now, proclaiming death caused by blood sucking insect.

He focused back to the matter at hand. A road map of Brookstone appeared in his mind as he calculated the quickest route to a shop. Braking hard, Dick swung into a left turn as a route materialised. The tyres chirped under acceleration out of the corner.

Aiming his vehicle directly at the front door of the store, Dick mounted the gutter and stopped on the footpath. He wasted no time exiting the vehicle. A surge of adrenalin had temporarily cured his arthritic hips as he pushed the car door open with a foot and ran into the general store. The tinkle of the small bell attached to the entrance door was lost as the police siren still wailed out front.

Dick yelled to the surprised shop owner, paralysed behind his counter. 'Where's your insect spray?'

The middle aged man pointed to an aisle, 'Just on the shelf to your left.'

Dick swept his body to the left and was confronted by six different brands of insect spray, in all different colours and sizes. 'Jesus Christ!' Dick pleaded to the Almighty again as he was momentarily confused by the selection.

He quickly snapped out of his indecision and grabbed two of the largest cans. 'Come with me.' Dick yelled back at the confused shop owner with such assertiveness that the owner climbed over his counter rather than go around it.

No sooner had Dick exited the store, he began to spray himself. He started with his boots and laces then worked his way up his overalls. By the time the shop owner made it outside, Dick was up to spraying his chest and arms.

Dick thrust the can of insect spray towards the shop owner. 'Spray my back. Start at my boots and work your way up.'

Dick turned and raised his arms out sideways, parallel to the ground, as the man did as he was told. The shop owner finished spraying Dick's back.

'Keep going until the can's empty,' Dick demanded as he started to rotate his body, still with arms held wide.

When the aerosol can was empty, Dick walked over to his vehicle and turned off the lights and siren. By this time a small crowd had gathered at the odd and amusing scene. Enjoying the free entertainment, strangers asked one another what was going on. All they could do in reply was shrug their shoulders and say, 'No idea.'

Ignoring the crowd, Dick then proceeded to fumigate the inside of his vehicle with the second can of spray. He sprayed the fabric seats and carpeted floor until that can was empty too.

Having calmed himself down, Dick approached the bemused shop owner. 'What do I owe you for the insect spray?' Dick casually asked as if nothing out of the ordinary had taken place.

The owner was at first at a loss for words, but then said, 'Why don't you come inside,' and indicated with a nod of his head towards the swelling crowd.

He entered the shop, followed by the owner who closed the door and turned the closed sign hanging from it to face outwards. Dick told the shop owner about the sequence of events that led him to his shop. By the end of the conversation, both men were laughing so hard they both started to cry. Dick's tears were helped by the stinging fumes of the insect spray that were wafting from his clothing.

It turned out that Dick had attended the store a year and a half ago following a break-in. His examination of the store was successful and an offender was arrested and convicted on the fingerprint evidence that Dick provided. The owner was still grateful and refused Dick's attempts to pay for the insect spray.

'I really want to pay for the spray,' Dick persisted.

'No, no. It's the least I can do. Besides, when I open the door again people will come in and just buy something to find out what all the fuss was about. Business will be booming.' The owner beamed a broad smile.

'And what are you going to tell them?' asked Dick with some trepidation.

'I don't know yet. But there will be no mention of fleas though,' laughed the shop owner again.

'You're a good man,' he replied and shook the owner's hand.

10AM

The fire brigade personnel were in the process of using their hydraulic cutting equipment to remove the roof of the crumpled four-wheel-drive. The cutting jaws slowly closed, causing the metal to twisted and pop, as they moved closer towards meeting.

Roslyn's body slumped to the right. Her head came to rest on the door's window sill. Her long black hair shone in the sunlight as it tumbled outside the vehicle and draped its side. A light breeze played through her hair, picking it up and tossing it gently, then allowing it to fall tenderly again.

Rowdy stood some distance away, mesmerised by the long flowing hair that was still full of life. He thought how beautiful it looked as it glittered under the sun and waved in the breeze.

For a brief moment, Rowdy fully detached himself from the reality of the scene. There was no sound of screeching metal as the cutting equipment continued to tear its way through. He could see the mouths of fireman moving as they yelled orders to one another, but no words registered in Rowdy's ears.

The scene before him was substituted with another. He could see the vision of a beautiful woman, sitting on a stool in front of a mirror. She was gently brushing her hair after running her fingers through its locks. She smiled as each soothing brush stroke filled her with a simple pleasure that can only be captured by immersing yourself into that single moment in time. 'Where are we up to, Rowdy?' Sergeant Wilkins had returned from the house.

Rowdy's illusion faded back into reality. He cursed himself for allowing that fleeting moment of emotion to penetrate his protective wall. He was again confronted by the noises around him. His eyes were again filled with the sight of Roslyn's horrendous facial injuries as a fireman gently pushed her back into an upright position.

'The government contractors are here,' Rowdy managed while throwing a thumb in the direction of the white van, then continued as a fireman threw a car door onto the ground, 'It looks like the boys are done.'

'We'll get her out of here then,' the Sergeant stated.

A genuinely concerned look appeared on Rowdy's face when he asked, 'How's everyone up at the house?'

'The kids are pretty good surprisingly. Dad's a mess. His in-laws are taking care of the kids at the moment.'

'Were you able to speak with the children about what happened?' asked Rowdy.

Sergeant Wilkins confirmed the assumption that they had made about the accident. 'I spoke with the eldest girl, Sophie. She's one tough kid. It's what we thought. Mum was rushing the kids down to the gate to catch the school bus when the car rolled.'

Rowdy continued his questioning, 'Will you need to speak with her again?'

'I don't see the point. I'll just include in my statement what Sophie told me. That should be sufficient for the Coroner's Brief,' replied Sergeant Wilkins.

'That's good. The kids have been through enough,' said Rowdy. 'The statement and photos provided by Crime Scene will explain the accident side of things.'

Never missing an opportunity to investigate, the old Sergeant's experience showed through when he said, 'While I was in the house I had a good look around and didn't see any alcohol or drug paraphernalia laying around. Anyway, the autopsy will cover if there was any contributing factor to the crash.'

The Crime Scene officer finished packing away his equipment. He stopped his vehicle next to the Sergeant and Rowdy as he drove down the driveway and leant through his open window. 'I'll leave you blokes with it.'

Sergeant Wilkins extended a handshake towards the officer. 'Thanks for all your help,' he said to soften the blow of his next question. 'When can I expect your statement?'

The officer laughed before replying, 'I'd have a better chance telling you who the next winner of the Melbourne Cup will be. Yours will be in the queue with about another fifty I've got to do.'

The Crime Scene section's work load was enormous. Like most specialist sections of the police force, they were under-staffed and over-worked. 'With a bit of luck the Coroner will dispense with an inquest,' Rowdy said optimistically.

'Here's hoping,' replied the officer who then continued to drive down the gravel driveway. A hand saluted out the open window as he departed.

Rowdy turned to the hovering funeral contractors and yelled, 'You're up, guys.'

Ricky pulled the last sheet of statement paper from the typewriter when the Station Sergeant approached. 'Are you done there, Ricky?' he asked.

He shuffled piles of paperwork into some sort of order. 'Finishing up now, sarge.'

'I'll get you to do charge room duty then. The Highway Patrol boys have just brought in an early pissy. He's blown point one-six.'

'That's a good drink for this time of the day,' said Ricky, impressed with the man's blood alcohol result.

'I've seen better,' replied the sergeant.

'Where's Frog?' Ricky asked, enquiring about the Station Officer whose role was to perform any charge duties for the shift.

'He's tied up taking a statement in my office.' A woman walked in wanting to report a domestic assault.'

Ricky knew the Station Sergeant did not have to explain his request to him. He knew even better not to argue the point.

'Righto,' Ricky replied. 'Give me a couple of minutes and I'll be right there.' As an afterthought and to test the boundaries, Ricky asked, 'The highway boys can't do the charging?'

The Station Sergeant showed restraint in having his request questioned. 'You know them, son. They don't mind catching them, but they don't like skinning them.' He turned and walked away; leaving Ricky in no doubt what was required of him.

Several minutes later, Ricky entered the Charge Room. He stood behind the high counter just as a Highway Patrol officer escorted a wobbly male into the room and placed him in the dock, located in one corner of the room. It was made from steel tubing, bolted to one wall then extended out nearly one and a half metres, before curving at right angles to attach to the adjacent wall. It basically created a small, confined area about waist height where prisoners stood while being charged. A prisoner could easily climb out of the dock if he had the inclination to do so, but most were resigned to their fate and waited patiently to be given bail.

'Morning John,' Ricky said to the Highway Patrol officer, as he closed the dock gate behind the offender.

Ricky turned to a fresh page in the charge book. 'A bit early in the morning for this, isn't it?'

'He found us.' The dishevelled man was now slumped over the dock rail, holding his head as he moaned. 'He nearly had a head on with us out on the highway.'

'One-sixty – that's a decent drink for this time of the day.'

'He had a big night,' John replied. 'He actually stopped drinking about three this morning. He slept some of it off in his car before he tried to weave his way home.'

Ricky turned his attention to the drunken man. 'Good morning, sir.' Ricky yelled in order to get his attention. The man moaned even louder as his hands clasped his head to prevent it from exploding from the pounding within.

'He's been no trouble so far,' John stated. 'I'll take his fingerprints and photograph if you like?'

Ricky was not going to reject the help. 'Thanks… that'll quicken things up.'

'Tombstone performed the breath test; said you blokes were busy.'

'I was wondering where he got to,' replied Ricky.

'Can I push the friendship and get you to search him while I enter up his property?'

'You know us highway boys… happy to help out,' John said, his voice heavy with irony.

Ricky stamped the charge book with the High Range Prescribed Concentration of Alcohol indictment, and wrote in the specific details of the offence. He then took three copies of the unconditional bail form from under the counter, slipped carbon paper between the sheets, and rolled them into the typewriter. Before he could start tapping away at the keys, *The Rock* walked into the charge room.

'Good morning gentleman,' he said in a low, unemotional voice that was laced with authority. The Rock was a large, barrel-chested man of immense strength. Each slow step was taken with purpose as he approached Ricky at the charge counter. His eyes darted from a face void of emotion as he continually assessed the room and everything around him. Many a man had been deceived by his slow movements, but when his eyes saw a need to react, the body did so with the speed of a thoroughbred racehorse and the grace of a ballroom dancer.

The Rock was actually a Senior Constable attached to the Chifley Highway Patrol. He carried out his duties with complete fairness to all that crossed his path by issuing a traffic infringement notice to everyone – no exceptions.

The Rock was the epitome of his nickname. He was a massive and immovable single block of solidly uniform stone that did not deviate for anyone, in particular, traffic offenders. His own mother could grovel at his feet, beg for mercy, and plead for leniency for having displayed an expired registration label on her car. Her fate, however, would be the same as all those who had gone before her. She would be met with that monotone voice of The Rock saying, 'Sorry, I cannot help you,' and then receive a fine.

'Good morning, Len,' Ricky greeted him cheerfully. 'Did you come to help out?'

'No,' said The Rock simply, leaving no room for confusion. 'I heard my offsider caught a pissy. I wish to use him as a research subject for my thesis.'

Behind The Rock's solid and stern façade was an agile and intelligent mind. He was currently completing a university doctorate in criminal studies.

'By all means,' replied Ricky, somewhat confused and turned to John. 'Any objection, John?'

'None at all,' he replied, and then added, a knowing smile spreading across his mouth, 'This should be very interesting.'

The Rock stood directly in front of the drunken man still slumped over the dock rail. 'You there,' he said tapping a thick muscular finger into the man's shoulder to gain his attention.

The man raised himself unsteadily to his full height. He clutched the dock rail firmly with both hands to steady his sway and politely slurred the words, 'Yessir.'

The Rock removed a piece of paper from a folder he was carrying and held it in front of the drunken man's face and demanded, 'What do you see?'

The drunken man looked through watery, bloodshot eyes at the ink blot held before him. His eyebrows rose as he forced his eyelids to open wider in his attempt to focus more clearly on the black stain.

'Shit!' the drunken man slurred in startled surprise that caused him to stagger back. 'That's how the missus looks when I get home after a night on the piss.'

The Rock returned the ink blot to his folder and then removed a second. He held it up to the man. 'What do you see?'

Still straining to see, the drunken man moved his weaving face closer towards the ink stained paper. He then jerked his head back with a look of horror etched upon it.

'Shit,' he slurred again. 'That's the mother-in-law after she's had a night on the piss.'

The drunken man retreated to the rear of the dock and wedged himself into the corner of the two walls. He raised his hands to safeguard his eyes as he attempted to block out the sight of the hideous form shown in the ink blot.

'Thank you, gentlemen,' The Rock said simply, as he returned the ink blot to his folder and left the room.

Dick had waited at the front of the general store for fifteen minutes with all four doors and the tailgate of his vehicle open to air it out. The wind now swirled like a cyclone through the car as he drove with all the windows down. He hated the wind, and detested days when you had to battle against it to perform basic tasks like walking in a straight line. He would definitely never drive with a window down, not even an inch. He loathed how it buffeted against his body, messed with his hair and throbbed into his eardrums. Today, however, he revelled in its caressing hands as it whirled through the cabin. Just as the wind is nature's way of cleansing the earth, Dick was using it to purge his clothing and the cabin of his vehicle of the sharp caustic odour of insect spray.

He raised a forearm to his nose and inhaled deeply the cotton sleeve of his overalls. The acrid smell of insect spray, laced with the scent of rotting human skin with an underlying bouquet of dog excrement, filled his nasal passage. Reeling from the smell, Dick leaned towards the open window and again revelled in the winds sweet caress as he made his way back to Brookstone Police Station for a shower and change of clothes.

10.30AM

In the charge room at Chifley Police Station, Ricky prepared to bail the drunken PCA offender when he was distracted by a commotion in the hallway just outside the room.

'Let me go!' an angry voice yelled. 'You're hurting me, yer bastards!' The young male burst through the door opening. He was attempting to thrash from side to side as he growled and snorted to be released. The man had each arm twisted and held firmly behind his back by two escorting police, who ignored his protests and threats of bodily harm.

Tony and Dean, who were part of the Chifley Police Target Action Group, escorted the man unceremoniously into the dock. The TAG officers were basically a pro-active arm of the general duties police. Where the GD's broadly reacted to crime, the TAG officers went out looking to prevent crime.

'Get in there and behave yourself,' Dean said, as he thrust the young man into the dock and closed the gate.

The drunken man, wedged in the corner, lifted his throbbing head as the angry young man jostled into him, still yelling obscenities towards his escorts. 'Keep it down boofhead, I'm trying to sleep,' he mumbled at the disturbance.

'Just wait until you're outside alone, mate. You won't know what hit you,' growled the angry young man towards Dean through clenched teeth, his cheek muscles pulsing with anger.

The drunken man came somewhat to life and slurred towards the young man, 'Let me give you some advice, son. Take it from a pro at this. There's a hard way and an easy way. You're doing it the hard way.' Having passed on his years of accumulated wisdom, the drunken man again leaned against the wall and closed his eyes.

Ignoring the solid advice, the angry youth continued his verbal threats. Dean had enough of the man's dribble. He walked back over to the dock, with vitriol clearly displayed in his eyes. He stood in front of the angry young man. Dean's muscular frame cleared that of the angry young man by a whole thirty centimetres. Leaning downwards, Dean placed his face into the young man's, their noses nearly touched, causing a quiver to pass across the man's bottom lip.

'Why put off until tomorrow what you can do today,' Dean snarled in a whisper. 'Give it your best shot,' he continued, and goaded the young man to strike out.

Dean's stare did not waver in intensity as he waited for a movement to indicate the young man's acceptance of his offer. Neither came. The angry young man just stood there, scared and not knowing what to do. He could no longer hold the police officer's stare and pulled away, diverting his eyes to his feet.

'Just what I thought,' said Dean softly, but obviously filled with the rage of a charging bull. 'You're nothing but a gutless little wimp, too wet behind the ears to be away from his mother.'

The drunken man began to chuckle. Through the haze of his insobriety, he appreciated the battle just fought between the experienced cop and a loud young buck. It was a battle that required no violence or bloodshed. It was a battle of wills that was clearly won by experience.

Dean turned away from the cowering young man and gave Ricky a wink. A wink that said, 'That's how it's done, son. Just call their bluff.'

'So, what have you got for me, Dean, now the show's over?'

'Fare evasion and assault,' Dean replied.

John had already photographed and fingerprinted the drunken man. 'I'll leave you with him,' he said to Ricky who only had to bail his PCA offender.

'More fish to catch I take it?' inquired Ricky as John made to leave.

'That's right. Looks like they're just starting to bite,' he replied and disappeared through the doorway.

Ricky returned his attention to Dean who was bent over the end of the charge counter writing up his notebook.

'So Dean, fare evasion and assault police is it?' Ricky asked, assuming that the angry young man had assaulted Dean and Tony during the arrest.

'No, he assaulted the taxi driver after refusing to pay his cab fare,' Dean said to clarify.

Ricky pushed aside the typewriter with its bail forms waiting to be completed and grabbed the property docket book.

'Tony, could you search your young man please?' asked Ricky

Tony quickly patted the young man down and removed a wallet and wristwatch from him. He placed the items on the counter top. Ricky opened the wallet and was surprised to find an amount of cash.

'There's one-hundred and twenty dollars here!' exclaimed Ricky when he finished counting. 'How much was the taxi fare?'

'Ten dollars,' Dean replied.

Tony had placed the young man back into the dock. Ricky gave him a look that said, 'You idiot. Why didn't you just pay the fare?'

The young man looked away from Ricky's inquiring gaze. He was now asking himself that same question.

Ricky completed the property docket entry, and then returned to the typewriter.

'I've just got to bail out our other mate here, and then I'll make a start on your bloke,' Ricky informed Dean. The drunken man was still happily dozing against the wall.

'Who was the victim anyway?' Ricky asked, as he tapped away at the typewriter keys.

'It was old Ronny Dart,' said Dean. 'He's been driving cabs here for fifty years.'

'He must have started with Cobb & Co,' Tony joked of the iconic transport company that made Chifley its headquarters in 1862.

'After refusing to pay the fare, our young mate belted Ronny and then tried to run away,' Dean explained. 'Some bike riders, who were stopped and having a morning coffee, saw the whole thing and actually grabbed him before he ran too far.'

The three police were then startled by a loud crack, followed by the thud of a body as it crumpled to the floor.

Tony and Dean, who had their backs to the dock, quickly turned around while Ricky looked up from the typewriter. Standing in the dock was the drunken man, rubbing the knuckles of his right hand. At his feet, curled on the floor unconscious, was the young man.

'Ronny's me mate,' spat the drunken man, with a slur. 'No-one hits Ronny and gets away with it.'

'Well… I'll be,' Tony said, impressed.

'Who said there's no justice in the world,' Dean casually added.

Ricky, concerned for the young man's welfare, walked to the dock and knelt down.

He reached through the lower rail and checked the man's pulse. 'He's still alive,' Ricky said thankfully. The last thing he needed was a *death in custody* investigation. particularly one when he was temporarily in charge of the man's safe custody.

'Should we get an ambulance?' Ricky asked the two more senior officers.

Dean shook his head, 'He'll be right,' he answered. 'Let's just enjoy the peace and quiet. Bail your old mate out, and then we'll splash some water on sleeping beauty.'

Ricky's concern now turned to himself, as he considered protecting his own butt. He pointed towards the drunken man who stood in the dock, extremely pleased with himself. 'Don't we have to charge him with assault?'

'Why complicate things,' Dean replied, unworried at what had happened. 'Anyway, did you see him assault anyone?'

'Well, no,' Ricky said hesitantly but honestly. The penny finally dropped as he realised to what Dean was alluding. 'I didn't see it,' he said now with confidence, something he could honourably swear to on oath.

'Neither did Tony or me. For all I know, he fainted,' said Dean.

Ricky opened the dock gate for the drunken man to sign his bail forms. After signing the necessary paperwork, Ricky escorted him to the front door of the police station. Ricky held the door open, but before the drunken man passed through he stopped and held out an open hand towards Ricky. Ricky shook the hand and was surprised at the firmness of the grip.

'Thank-you,' said the drunken man, grateful for not being charged with assault. 'Like I said, there's an easy way and a hard way.'

'Anytime,' Ricky smiled back with true meaning. 'Can I get you a lift home?'

'No, I need to sober up more before facing the missus,' said the drunken man, releasing his vice-like grip on Ricky's hand.

Ricky watched the man stagger from one edge of the concrete path to the other, then stumble when the toe of his shoe caught a crack. Ricky could only wonder how on earth he had managed to land a punch square on the angry young man's jaw.

'Don't drive,' Ricky called out before re-entering the police station.

Dick could already feel the warm, cleansing shower on his body as he counted down the minutes till his arrival back at Brookstone Police Station. He was determined not the let the house of horrors effect the rest of his day. After all, it was the one and only job he had for the day, and it was now behind him. Its images, however, regularly flashed through his mind as the wafting odour still filled the car and could be tasted on the back of his throat. He could still feel his skin tingle. As much as he told himself that it was all in his mind, he could not help but renew his efforts to scratch to rid the vermin that attacked his mind.

'No way,' Dick said to himself as he recognised a bicycle rider approaching him. 'I don't need that grubby piece of shit right now.'

There's a saying that if it looks like a duck, quack likes a duck, then it's a duck. The police had a similar saying - If it looks like shit and smells like shit, then its shit. No truer saying applied to the grub on the push bike. Leslie Scott Tower. It was as though the house of horrors had sent for re-enforcements to play with Dick's mind.

Tower rode his push bike on the wrong side of the road. He was travelling towards Dick head-on, the bike's wheels following the painted white edge line. Tower sat arrogantly upright as he peddled shirtless and without a helmet. He possessed that insolent body language which impelled most people who saw him to want to hit him rather than talk to him.

Tower was actually one of Dick's best customers. He was a hopeless, drug-addicted, dole bludger who resorted to robbery and theft of any kind to pay for his habit. Dick had caught him no less than seven times by matching his fingerprints to a scene.

To contemplate wearing gloves to his crimes was about as far from his thoughts as getting a job and making an honest living. There were three occasions that his DNA had been linked to a crime. He could not help but discard a cigarette butt inside a home, or cut himself breaking a window and leave copious amounts of blood to identify him by. He was just a hopeless druggie, and a less than capable thief.

There can be a funny bond that can form between police and offenders. A bond based on mutual respect for the way each individual ply their trade. If your chosen career is to be a thief, at least try and be a good one. The same as any police officer should try to excel at what they do. It becomes a game of cat and mouse, with each side prepared to lose sometimes, but to do all in their power to win.

There was no such bond between Dick and Leslie Scott Tower. It was only two weeks ago that Tower had overdosed and was found lying in the gutter with a bottle of stolen prescription pills next to him. After being rushed to hospital and revived, he woke violently; striking out at the nurses and ambos who were trying to save his life. Dick happened to be nearby when the hospital requested police assistance with the violent patient.

He was more than happy to help restrain Tower while a nurse fed a large tube through his nose and down into his stomach. It was a satisfying sight to see him squirm in pain and discomfort as the tube was fed deeper inside him. A large syringe, filled with saline, was then attached to the tube and its contents forced into Tower's stomach. Dick couldn't help snigger out loud as the syringe was then used like a suction pump to suck out the contents of the stomach. The whole time, Tower struggled against his restraints and yelled in agony. Dick remembered the nurses being horrified at his lack of compassion for the poor misguided soul who had been let down by society.

He will never forget the look on the nurses' faces when the procedure was concluded and asked, 'Can't we do it just one more time?'

The distance between Dick and Tower continued to close.

'Why did some do-gooder have to ring triple zero that day?' Dick asked himself as he fixated on Tower. 'The ambos should have left the trash in the gutter for the street sweeper to collect, and dump it with all the rest of society's waste,' he continued to say to himself.

The anger inside Dick began to boil as he considered all the time and money that had been expended on this one parasite. His inner dialogue kept asking questions, 'How many people could have been put through an apprenticeship, or university, on the money spent keeping this low life alive?' his mind ranted. 'If it had been spent on medical research, how many lives could have been saved where the patient didn't choose their illness.'

Dick's mind was now completely obsessed with the bike rider. His body tensed and his grip on the steering wheel firmed as his palms began to sweat. He could feel his temples throb, and hear each beat of his heart as his own unanswered questions kept raging in him, 'How many times has he been caught and sent to gaol? But here he is, back out again to continue his felonious ways - at least until he is caught again, and treated to three meals a day at our expense.'

The expanse of roadway between the two narrowed further. Dick's thoughts now became more irrational. Thoughts that once would never have occurred to him now seemed logical and sensible. 'This is my chance,' he said mutely with sudden realisation.

All Dick saw now was a target to vent all his neurotic frustrations on. He was in the protection and safety of nearly two tonne of vehicle. Tower, on the other hand, was exposed and vulnerable on his bicycle.

'All it will take is a minor steering adjustment to the left,' Dick's mind rationalised. 'I can't help it if a drug affected cyclist swerves in front of me.' Dick now mouthed the words that entered his mind in a scaringly calm and self-convincing voice, 'An early death is just what he deserves.' The pounding drum in his head was like the Pausarius on a Roman Galley, who quickened his drum beat to mark the oar stroke of its rowers. The distance between Dick and Tower decreased rapidly. The truncheon beating inside his head grew louder as Dick reached ramming speed. The bonnet at the front of his vehicle was now a bronze bow-ram, ploughing on to strike its target.

Dick's fingers extended out from the steering wheel when he was within six metres of Tower. They curled back tightly now, as Dick braced his body with only four metres separating the two opposing forces.

'Do it,' the voice yelled in Dick's head. The steering wheel twitched to the left.

Rowdy and Sergeant Wilkins stood to one side as the funeral contractors positioned their trolley near the opening of the four-wheel-drive created by the fire brigade. A black body-bag lay on the gurney and was unzipped by one of the men. The thick plastic parted like the mouth of a whale shark, ready to devour whatever came its way.

'Just sing out if you need a hand, fellas,' said Sergeant Wilkins obligingly. Rowdy was just thinking how unusually helpful his old Sergeant was being to assist with the grizzly task of removing Roslyn from the vehicle, when Sergeant Wilkins continued, 'And I'll get my offsider here to give you some help.'

Ricky gave his Sergeant a sharp look.

'What?' Sergeant Wilkins replied innocently. 'Every job needs a supervisor,' he continued, and made a point of looking at the crown and stripes insignia that decorated his shoulders.

The two contractors, who had each donned a pair of disposable overalls and latex gloves, positioned themselves. On the count of three they lifted in unison. They strained under Roslyn's dead weight and barely managed to lift her clear of the seat.

Roslyn's arms were extended up and out to the side as the contractor tried to lift higher. He resorted to standing on his toes to gain the extra height as his upper body strength neared its limit. Roslyn was as flexible as a rag doll. The second contractor faced a similar problem when he lifted her legs. The knees initially just rose up as her legs pivoted at the hips. Fortunately, the raised driving position of the large four-wheel-drive was at a similar height to the gurney. Their movement became more of a drag than a lift as they slewed the body sideways.

Roslyn was bent in two as her knees lifted into her chest. Her head flopped forward and wobbled from side to side as the contractors took shuffling sideways steps. They then swung the body towards the waiting gurney and grunted from the exertion. Roslyn's inert body flopped down. Her arms escaped over each side of the gurney while one knee remained propped in the air momentarily before falling to the side.

'It doesn't look like she wants to go in, does it?' the old Sergeant said to no one in particular.

'Just letting you know now, fellas,' Rowdy quipped to the contractors as they organised the flailing parts of the body back onto the bed. 'I'm not going to go without a fight either.'

As a contractor was tucking the arms into the body bag, Rowdy noticed a chain bracelet on one wrist.

'Before you zip her up, I'll just grab the jewellery she's wearing,' said Rowdy to the contractor, who had just pushed a leg in and taken hold of the zipper.

Rowdy snapped on a pair of latex gloves from his PPE kit fitted to his appointments belt. He slid his hand into the body bag and lifted Roslyn's limp, right arm to remove the bracelet. He also noticed a gold coloured necklace that was dulled with blood. He gently brushed aside some blood matted hair and swivelled the necklace around until the latch was at the front. He released the clasp, and handed the jewellery to Sergeant Wilkins, who entered their details into his police notebook.

Rowdy then pulled out the left arm. A wedding band sat snugly on Roslyn's ring finger. Rowdy gave a gentle pull on the ring, but the only movement was the skin around it which stretched with each tug. Rowdy tried wiggling the ring, but it wouldn't pass over the knuckle.

Rowdy happened to glance inside the four-wheel-drive. A white plastic tube on the floor under the brake pedal caught his eye. 'What's that on the floor, Sarge?' he said, pointing towards the tube.

'Thirty-plus sunscreen,' replied the sergeant, as he lifted it from the floor.

'That'll do,' said Rowdy and held out his hand to take the tube.

Rowdy squeezed a liberal amount of the white greasy cream onto the ring and then rubbed it into Roslyn's skin.

'I think sun burn is the least of her troubles at the moment, Rowdy,' Sergeant Wilkins joked.

'Hopefully it will give enough lubrication…' Rowdy paused as he wiggled and turned the ring again, '…to slip the ring off,' he continued triumphantly, holding the ring between his thumb and index finger and peered through its centre.

'You might want to clean that off before you give it back to the family,' said Rowdy to his Sergeant and handed him the slimy wedding band.

11AM

'Forensics 229, Forensics 229,' came the police radio operators call.

Dick flinched, startled by the amplified voice calling his vehicle call sign. More importantly, it startled his thought process out of its neurosis. Just like an electric charge brings a fibrillating heart back into rhythm, the sharp sound coming from the radio realigned his thought process back into reality.

Refusing the demands of his inner demons, Dick flinched back into the present moment and so too did the steering wheel. The minute turn of the steering wheel back to centre was enough to alter the vehicle's collision course. Dick passed the bicycle with only millimetres between it and the side mirror of his car. All Dick saw, as the bike passed in a blur, were two white eyes as large as dinner plates.

Dick instantly swivelled in his seat to look behind him but then just as quickly faced the front again. He glanced up at his rear vision mirror and saw that the bicycle behind him had developed a severe wobble. The erratic push bike veered right, towards the gravel verge that lined the roadway's edge. Its rider no longer peddled but had his legs splayed out to the sides in mid-air as the bicycle wobbled violently beneath him.

Tower slowly regained control of the wayward bike and avoided an untimely dismount onto the gravel. All Tower could do now, as he turned his head and looked over his shoulder at the departing police car, was raise his left hand high into the air and give the receding vehicle and Dick a middle finger salute.

Sweat that beaded on Dick's forehead now trickled down his face. He panted for breath as if he had just finished a strenuous workout.

He was confused to the point that he had to quickly look around to recognise landmarks and reorientate himself.

As he regained his bearings, the reality of what had just happened flooded back to him. 'Jesus, I could have killed him!' Dick said out loud and was then suddenly overcome with a wave of nausea that threatened to project from his mouth. Dick swallowed hard as the radio operator called again. Dick could see Brookstone Police Station in the distance as he acknowledged the call.

'Thanks 229. We have a request from Kingstown Crime Scene to attend the Kingstown Morgue and fingerprint a deceased from your area,' informed the radio operator.

'Who will be the fingerprint expert to see, radio?' Dick asked, still tasting the bile in his throat.

The fingerprinting of deceased persons for identification purposes was a job for a qualified fingerprint expert, not a SOC officer like Dick. He wrongly assumed he would meet up with one of the experts at the morgue.

'Sorry 229,' replied the operator. 'No experts are available. The request has come from the Crime Scene Supervisor who said you have had experience and training in this field.'

Dick paused as he considered the legalities of this request. Basically, all he would be doing is obtaining the fingerprints. The actual identification process would still have to be performed by a fingerprint expert, which can occur any time after the prints are obtained.

Satisfied that there could be no legal issue to later compromise an investigation, Dick replied, 'Copy radio. I'm assuming it's the drowning victim recovered yesterday?'

'That's correct 229,' confirmed the operator.

Dick acknowledged, and returned the radio handpiece to its cradle.

'Just what I need,' he mumbled as he drove past Brookstone Police Station.

His shower and change of clothes would have to wait. He turned left onto the Great North Highway and started his journey south to Kingstown.

Dick was aware that yesterday afternoon, a body had been fished out of a nearby lake. It was a popular camping and fishing site, surrounded by spectacular peaked mountains that rolled gracefully into the water. The lake was filled with bass, and other aquatic life, that provided anglers with hours of enjoyment and frustration as they dangled their tempting lures. Power boats and jet skis thrashed the surface with skiers, wake boarders, and tubes filled with laughing children in tow.

It was a peaceful and picturesque location for most; however, three days previously, a middled aged man had attended the lake to go fishing from his canoe. The alarm was raised when he failed to return home. His unattended canoe was found blown aground on a remote bank, away from the main camping area. A search of the shallows revealed no trace of the man and it was feared he lay one hundred and sixty metres down in the depths of the lake.

Three days later, a holidaying fisherman caught the catch of the day when he noticed something bobbing in the water. At first he thought it was driftwood and manoeuvred his vessel closer with the purpose of removing the hazard it posed to boating. As the fisherman neared the flotsam, its form took on the shape of a lifeless body, floating face down with arms and legs dangling beneath the water.

After falling from his canoe and drowning, the victim sank to the murky depths as soon as the air in his lungs was replaced with water.

The body had now ballooned to twice its size. Gases had built up in the stomach and chest cavity as the body began to decay. As the levels of carbon dioxide, methane, and hydrogen sulphide accumulated in the body, it became buoyant again and caused the body to return topside.

The torso usually bloats more than the limbs and head as it contains the greatest number of bacteria which produce the gases. As such, the torso will usually rise to the surface first, dragging the limbs below it, which is why the body will normally float facing down.

When the fisherman righted the body, the full extent of the tragedy was exposed which caused him to stumble backwards, tripping over tackle boxes, rocking the boat and threatening to capsize it.

After three days of immersion, the fish and yabbies had feasted on the decaying flesh. Wherever skin was exposed, the leftover signs of the banquet were evident, as flesh was torn, and dangled in shreds from the body. The eyes were missing and the face unrecognisable in its swollen and tattered state. This is the sight that now awaited Dick.

It is a fair bet that the person who fell out of the canoe and drowned three days ago, is the same person found floating, but a positive identification was still required. As the body was not in a fit state to have family members perform a visual identification, the ID had to be undertaken by different means. The next practical and cost effective means to do this is by fingerprint identification. Even if the deceased did not have a criminal record with his fingerprints in the system, fingerprint experts or a SOC Officer would attend the home of the suspected dead person. They would attempt to develop fingerprints on surfaces or objects inside the home. If one of these prints could be matched to the victim, then this was sufficient identification for the Court.

The other consideration that police investigating had to face was, could another person have drowned, or even been murdered and dumped in the lake? As the answer to this question is always yes, it was imperative that a positive identification of any deceased was made.

Lindsay Crisp slammed the lid closed on the car boot and turned to walk towards the driver's door. 'Don't close that yet,' his wife's voice came as she rushed down the back steps of their farm house.

'I thought we had everything packed,' Lindsay replied as he noticed his wife carrying another small bag.

'I've just got this one last bag to put in,' Lynda replied.

'We're only going for one night remember, not the whole week.'

'You never know what a girl might need in the big smoke,' said Lynda, excited about their trip to Sydney to pick up their son. 'I can't pick Mark up looking like I just removed my arm from a cow's rear end, can I?'

Lindsay rolled his eyes as his wife placed the bag into the boot that he again opened. 'There won't be room to pick him up if you keep filling the car with all this stuff.'

Lynda ignored her husband's remark. Instead, she chastised him for his footwear. 'You're not wearing those boots, I hope?'

'What's wrong with them?' Lindsay protested with his own question.

'Just look at them,' Lynda said as they both now starred down at Lindsay's scuffed and worn work boots. 'And they smell like cow dung,' she added, turning up her nose.

'I can't smell anything,' said Lindsay, knowing full well that he would not be allowed to leave the farm with them on. He could feel his wife's eyes boring into him. 'I'll just go change them then,' he succumbed with a loving smile.

'Well, hurry up then. We don't want to be late,' remarked Lynda, not knowing how prophetic those words would be.

Lindsay returned to the house and disappeared through the back door. It was the same every time they went somewhere. He could be just ducking into town to pick up some supplies and his wife would make him change something he was wearing. The request to change was always followed by his wife remarking, 'It's inappropriate,' and Lindsay would always reply, 'Yes, dear,' just to keep life simple.

Lindsay reappeared and returned to the car wearing a pair of RM's that looked like they had just come out of the box.

'There. That's more appropriate now, isn't it?' said Lynda triumphantly with a nod of her head.

'Come on then, it's time to get the boy,' Lindsay said as he opened the car door for his wife. As he closed the door behind her he mumbled to himself, '… and give me a break.'

Their car made its way down the driveway with a tail of dust left drifting across the paddocks. Lindsay eyed the fence line as he drove, checking for broken strands of wire. The last thing he wanted while he was away from the property was for cattle to get out onto the roadway or into the vegetable gardens.

He stopped the car at the entrance to the property and checked the main road for traffic. He was about to turn out when his wife's arm darted across the centre console and placed a hand on his leg to stop him.

'Should I just duck back and get that nice green coat of mine? It could turn cold,' she said.

Lindsay paused a moment, then asked, 'Do you have a coat already packed?'

'Well, yes,' replied Lynda, 'But….'

Lindsay cut her off. 'Well, you can only wear one at a time, so the one in the boot will do.'

Lindsay turned left. Their long drive to Sydney was under way.

Ricky returned to the charge room after seeing the drunken man from the premises. Dean and Tony were attempting to prop the still unconscious angry young man into a sitting position.

'How is he?' Ricky asked.

'He'll be okay,' replied Dean. He gently started to shake the angry young man into consciousness. 'Come on, son. That's enough time spent in the land of nod… back to reality.'

The booming voice of the Station Sergeant entered the room.

'What's happened here?' he demanded, as he stood and observed two of his officers huddled in the dock with the offender.

Startled by the voice, Ricky turned with a jerk to see the Station Sergeant approach from behind. Ricky's face drained of all colour as the towering figure filled him with dread.

'Well, you see sarge…' Ricky started to say hesitantly.

'Everything is fine sarge,' Deans unwavering voice now replied. 'He just fainted.'

A disbelieving look clearly showed on the Sergeant's face. 'What caused him to faint?' he inquired with a raised eyebrow.

Without hesitating and remaining straight faced, Dean said, 'I can only assume it was the overpowering grief that his criminal transgression has caused him. It has probably filled him with such crushing remorse, coupled with the overwhelming reality of the consequences that now await him, that must have caused him to faint.'

'You're full of shit,' said the Station Sergeant accusingly. 'What's that red welt on the side of his face?'

'Must have hit his face on the way down, sarge,' Dean again replied without hesitation.

The Sergeant now turned an inquisitive gaze towards Ricky and Tony, 'What about you two then?' he asked.

'Yep, fainted sarge,' Tony replied with conviction.

'Fainted,' Ricky said, less convincingly.

The three officers waited in various states of nervousness for their supervisor to respond. They all breathed again when the Station Sergeant ordered, 'Make sure there's a record made of it then.'

He then vanished from the room as he saw the young man coming to. He did not want to be in the room when the angry young man started telling a different story. The Charge Officer, who Ricky was relieving for, walked into the charge room. 'Good timing, Frog,' Ricky said with relief. 'This one is all yours to charge.'

'What's this mess on the floor then?' Frog asked as he indicated towards the young man.

'Dean and Tony will fill you in. I'm out of here,' said Ricky and hastily left the room.

Rowdy was back in Benstown, sitting in his Highway Patrol office. He was in the process of typing up the identification statement from his notebook, when he paused and reached for the telephone. He decided to ring his wife in case she heard something on the news reports about the accident. If the reports mentioned the location and a school bus being involved, she would be beside herself with worry.

'Hi,' Rowdy said cheerfully as his wife answered. He anticipated his wife's first response and was not disappointed.

'No, nothing is wrong,' Rowdy sighed. It did not occur to him why the tragic death of a mother failed to count as being something wrong. In Rowdy's world, this was just another everyday occurrence. If it had not happened at Bowen, then it would have happened somewhere else. In his world, people died all the time.

'I just wanted to let you know that Sharon, the bus driver, came across an accident when she was doing her rounds this morning,' Rowdy managed to say before being interrupted.

'The kids are fine,' he reassured his wife. 'They thought it was all very exciting,' he said as the next question came.

'A woman rolled her car,' he answered, not wanting to give to many details. He would tell his wife a more detailed version when he got home, but would spare her the details of the horrific injuries. He always kept that to himself. It was sufficient for him to say that the person had died. The extent of injuries did not make them any more or less dead, so he always spared the gruesome bits.

'Yes, I'm fine too,' Rowdy said, as he replied to the question from the other end of the phone line.

Rowdy, like a lot of other people, always said he was fine – even if he was not. He could see no point in burdening others with his problems. After all, what could they do to help, he wrongly thought. The other side of the coin was that if he admitted to someone else he was not fine, then that would be admitting to himself he had problems. He was not ready to admit that truth. Not yet anyway. His lone battle with his inner self was not over just yet. He still felt that he could control the numbness that was slowly consuming him. After all, he was not going to let the *bastards* win.

'No, I won't forget about picking the kids up,' he replied, and to save the next question being asked, said, '…and I haven't forgotten about tonight either.'

'Okay. Bye. Love you too,' he said before hanging up the phone.

Rowdy completed typing his ID statement and took it to Sergeant Wilkins, who was preparing the Coroner's Brief. 'Anything else I can do for you Sarge?' Rowdy asked as he stood in the Station Sergeant's office.

'No, nothing else. Thanks for all you help, though.'

'Anytime.'

'You'd better get back to whatever it was you were supposed to be doing today,' adding sarcastically, 'I'd hate to interfere with all that important work you highway blokes do.'

'Top priority today is seat belts,' Rowdy replied.

'Just think. If Roslyn had a seat belt on, she might be alive now.'

That was just one of the many 'what ifs' you could ask in any situation. In the end, it was never just one thing that lead to a tragedy. It was always a series of events, circumstances and decisions. It was unfortunate we could not go back and change the past. The future was primarily based on the unknown, which only left one thing that we could control – now.

As for Rowdy, he was spending less time enjoying the now because his mind was spending more time trapped in the gloom of the past, and anxiety about the future.

11.30AM

Dick leaned across and turned the volume of the police radio down before raising the volume on the commercial radio to a level that could be clearly heard outside the vehicle, let alone inside.

Since the near miss with Tower and the bicycle, Dick's mind had been consumed with replays. He hoped the music that pulsed through the speakers would distract his thoughts back on track and into the present. It was only partially working… Dick would start off humming the lyrics of every new song that played but the loud music would soon fade to a distant background noise.

He turned the volume up even louder until he could feel the music pulse through the air. Again the song would drift into the atmosphere, as muted as if he was wearing ear muffs.

The replays kept making their way to the forefront of his thoughts. He still argued over the worthlessness of the bicycle rider, failing to see how similar Tower was to him. Dick's traumatised mind was a direct result of his experiences and circumstances, as was Tower's criminal behaviour. Both men, who were on opposite sides of the coin, were on similar slippery slopes of life.

Dick started to reminisce about how this type of person may have been dealt with twenty-one years ago, when he was first in the job. He could now sympathise with those more senior police he had worked with in his younger days, as they themselves battled with the frustration of dealing with the same offenders, over and over again.

He vividly recalled working one late shift out west. It was the middle of winter where the temperature could drop into the minuses. Back in those days, Dick was rostered on night work from eleven to seven-thirty the following morning for seven nights straight.

On one particular roster, Dick and his more senior offsider were continually called to disturbances by one particular youth. The boy was never doing anything too serious, nor harming anyone else, but kept making a nuisance of himself around the town, fuelled by his level of intoxication. On the third successive night, about two in the morning, he was stumbling down the main street, kicking over garbage bins. Dick's offsider had enough of the young idiot but chose not to follow formal procedures. The youth would more likely be issued a paltry punishment at court, if anything at all.

Instead, the youth was unceremoniously tossed into the cage of the police truck, and Dick told to drive out of town. It was sixty kilometres between towns in either direction, with nothing but forest in between. Dick's offsider made sure that the ventilation flaps on the cages vinyl cover were secured in the open position. The sub-zero breeze would whistle through the cage like an Arctic blizzard as they drove at one-hundred kilometres an hour into the darkness. Dick was also told to hit as many potholes as possible and frequently swerve harshly, as if avoiding kangaroos that leapt into his path. The ride in the cage was uncomfortable, to say the least.

When halfway to the next town, Dick was told to pull over and stop. The rear door of the cage was opened and the near frozen and bruised youth gingerly staggered out. Dick's offsider then gave the youth a verbal dressing down and finished by saying, 'And when you get back to town, you play by our rules.' Dick and his senior colleague then drove back into town, leaving the youth abandoned by the roadside in the frigid temperatures. The result – the youth never gave any more trouble.

If he was ever spoken to by Dick or the other officer after that, his replies were usually a respectful, 'Yes sir', and 'No sir.'

'Thank Christ he didn't freeze to death or get hit by a car as he made his long journey back into town,' Dick thought to himself now. If anything was tried like that these days, Dick would be charged and given the sack. The idea still appealed to him, though, as he was buoyed by visions of that grub, Tower, standing freezing in the dark on a desolate highway.

The music started to register in Dick's ear again as he scrambled his way out of the depths of the past. He was making good headway on his journey to Kingstown Morgue. The frightening thing was not what awaited Dick at the morgue, but his inability to remember driving through the last town. As his mind had wondered back in time, so too did his concentration. The images that appeared before his eyes were not of the road ahead but the sights from the past. It was pure luck that there was not an accident.

Seeing how the music failed to work, Dick again wound down the car's window. He hoped the breeze would freshen his mind and sharpen his concentration. It would also help freshen up the car's interior, along with his clothing, that still reeked of insect spray.

His thoughts now turned more positive as he considered how he could improve his day. The trip to Kingstown could actually work in his favour. His elderly father was currently in a hospital, close to the morgue. After finishing his business at the morgue, he could visit his father before returning to Brookstone. With that thought, Dick managed to smile.

'Hi, Rowdy,' Bryan said happily, as he strode into the Benstown Highway Patrol office to commence his shift.

'Morning guys,' replied Rowdy, looking up from his computer screen to see Bryan walk into the room, followed by Baz.

'I thought you would be out on the road and a ticket book filled with seatbelt breaches,' Baz said to Rowdy.

Rowdy stretched back in his chair and rubbed his eyes to remove the glare of the computer monitor. 'I've had a bit of a delay this morning,' he replied, and went on to update the two officers about the morning's accident.

'How unlucky is that,' Bryan remarked of Roslyn's death.

Baz took a positive view of the events and said, 'But how lucky are the kids.'

'Very lucky. Only a few scrapes and bruises,' agreed Rowdy.

'So,' Bryan said to try and lighten the mood. 'You ready to do some real work now?' he asked, placing his work bag onto another desk. 'Enough of this playing with dead people, we've got lives to save out there.'

'Didn't your mother ever tell you not to play with dead people, Rowdy?' Baz added.

Rowdy ignored their comments and turned the conversation to the seatbelt enforcement they were required to perform. 'I thought we could team up for an hour or so. Baz, you can spot while Bryan and I'll do the writing.'

It was common practice to stand an officer near a roadway in a position that gave them clear vision of oncoming traffic. They didn't have to hide, they just had to stand on the footpath and mingle in with the other pedestrians walking past. A passing motorist would rarely see them. The officer would spot anyone not wearing a seatbelt, and call, via portable radio to police positioned further down the road. These police would then stop the offending driver and issue a traffic infringement notice for the offence.

'How come I'm always the spotter?' Baz complained.

'Where do you want to work it?' Bryan asked, ignoring the whine from Baz.

'There's that good spot in the sixty zone on the highway,' suggested Rowdy.

'The one near Batikin Park?' Bryan said to clarify the location.

'That's the one,' confirmed Rowdy. 'Traffic is usually a bit congested there and doing well under sixty to make it easier to spot and stop.'

Bryan and Baz liked the location.

'That's settled then,' Rowdy said and rose from his chair. 'Oo...ah,' he groaned as he straightened and a sharp pain shot up his back.

'What's wrong with you?' inquired Bryan.

It was the first time Rowdy had felt the pain today. He placed a hand to his lower back and arched backwards slightly to stretch out the discomfort. 'Just a bit of a twinge every now and then after getting knocked down the other night.'

'What happened?' asked Bryan, more interested in a story than Rowdy's discomfort.

Rowdy continued to massage his back. 'I backed up the GD's at a brawl at one of the pubs,' Rowdy started to explain.

'I hope you didn't rush to get there?' Bryan asked, but meant it more as a statement. 'It's much easier to pick the pieces up after it's done and dusted.' The pieces, that Bryan mentioned, were a reference to the combatants involved.

'The main battle had been fought and won by the time we got there,' continued Rowdy. 'The main participants had managed to settle their differences, without causing major damage to one another, and had dissolved into the crowd.'

'So how did you end up getting injured?' Baz asked with concern, but then added, 'Strain your back getting out of the car, did you?'

'You know what a crowd of drunken idiots is like. Push soon turns to shove once the initial entertainment has finished,' Rowdy continued to explain. 'This one particular foul- mouthed, drunken young lady started inciting the crowd to turn on the coppers, so I arrested her.'

'She get the better of you, Rowdy?' Baz laughed.

'No, but she did try to bite me, which I took offence to,' Rowdy said and inspected his arm for the teeth marks that had now faded. 'After I finally restrained her, I started to escort her towards the GD's truck. Someone then ran out of the crowd behind me at full gallop and dropped their shoulder into my back.'

'Did you see who it was?' asked Bryan.

Rowdy shook his head. 'No, I was knocked straight to the ground. By the time I got back up, the person was long gone, back into the safety of the crowd.'

'You're lucky you weren't hurt more seriously,' Baz remarked with genuine concern.

'The girl I was holding broke my fall. I didn't let go of her the whole time and she just happened to fall between me and the bitumen,' Rowdy said with a deceptive smile spreading across his face.

Police work was often a contact sport. While Rowdy's good nature did not wish harm on anyone, he was inwardly satisfied that the girl had suffered in some small way for her actions. He did not know it now but she would later plead not guilty to her offensive language and conduct charges. In order to receive leniency from the court, her legal aid solicitor would produce photos of the bruises and other injuries she received that night, and claim police brutality as the cause. The Magistrate would find her guilty of the charges but no penalty would be handed down and Rowdy would later be subjected to an internal affairs investigation.

'Did you file a hurt on duty report for your back injury?' Bryan asked, in a more serious tone.

'It's just a twinge,' replied Rowdy.

In Rowdy's fourteen year career, he had never submitted an HOD claim. It was not because he had never been injured at work; he just saw the bumps and bruises along the way as part of the game.

In the end, Rowdy's biggest injury would be the one he failed to see. It was an injury that did not show up on any X-ray or scan.

'Enough of this idle chitchat,' said Rowdy to the other two officers. 'Suit up and let's make a start.'

With Rowdy's encouragement, Bryan and Baz left in the direction of the change room. Rowdy returned to his computer and saved the statement he had been working on. After all, his backlog of work, and then some would still be there tomorrow.

It was tradition at Chifley Police Station for everyone to down-tools at ten am and congregate in the meal room for morning tea. Actually, it was not really tradition, but a request from the Chief Inspector, who ran the station. All the different sections were required to be there, including administration staff. It was the boss's way of keeping everyone functioning as a team. It also allowed him to judge what morale was like. The gathering also doubled as an intelligence swapping venue, for all that important information police kept in their heads and didn't write down, to formally share with others. It was surprising the number of times that an officer would make a passing comment about someone they were looking for, only to have another pipe up to inform them that they had crossed paths with that same person recently and could give address details of where to find them.

Sometimes however, operational duties had to be given priority over the boss's morning tea break. Today was one of those days. Ricky, along with many of the other staff from the different sections, had missed today's morning tea. Ricky finally found time for a break.

'A coffee, Tombstone?' Ricky asked.

'No thanks.' Tombstone had managed to have his morning tea break after performing the breath analysis for the highway patrol.

Ricky got up from his desk where he had started to type up some P40 Incident Reports from the previous day. They were the mundane stuff. Lost property reports, a gnome stolen from someone's garden and a malicious damage to a letter box. This was the real side of police work. He made his way towards the muster room door, but before he could pass through it, the Station Sergeant filled its frame.

'Ricky,' he said with his trademark boom. 'Just the man I was looking for.'

Ricky didn't have time to reply, or even think about what he had done wrong, when the Station Sergeant continued, 'I forgot to mention to you this morning, before you raced off and did that deaden, Internal Affairs will be here at twelve-thirty to interview you.'

The blood drained from Ricky's face at the mention of the Police Internal Investigation Branch.

'IA, what do they want?' Ricky asked apprehensively.

'It's from a complaint made from a gentleman you and Henry charged with goods in custody about eight months ago.'

'What's the complaint?' Ricky inquired with surprise.

'He claims one of you assaulted him,' came the unexpected reply.

'I've never assaulted anyone in my life,' said Ricky adamantly.

The Station Sergeant gave a deep throaty chuckle. 'Tell that to the judge.' He could still be heard chuckling as he left and made his way back to his own office.

'Eight months ago,' Ricky said, as he turned to face Tombstone. 'How am I supposed to remember what happened eight months ago?'

Tombstone gave him an inquiring look and asked, 'You made detailed notes at the time?'

'I'd only been in the job a few months. I was lucky if I could even write back then,' he said, remembering how everything was such a big learning curve when he first started.

'You'll be okay,' Tombstone replied. 'It'll all come back to you when they start asking questions.'

'I hope so.' Ricky felt the first twist of his stomach from nerves.

Tombstone's face was serious. 'If it doesn't go well and they lock you up, can I have that nice pen set you keep in your pigeon hole?'

Ricky's bowels now started to feel loose.

12 NOON

Rowdy parked his Highway Patrol car against the kerb. He activated his red and blue emergency beacons, to better advertise his presence. He also turned on the rear facing LED message board that formed part of the integrated roof bar. Of the twenty-five pre-programmed messages that could be displayed, Rowdy selected 'Buckle Up' from the menu, and sent it streaming across the bright red display.

'That should stop people whinging about us hiding,' Rowdy said to Bryan, who had arrived after dropping Baz off.

'If they can't see that, then their driving with their head up their arse,' Bryan commented, pulling a high visibility reflective vest over his head. 'There, that should give them a good enough target to hit when I walk in front of them.'

'If you're not bright enough for them to see, you're certainly a big enough target,' said Rowdy, as he watched Bryan attempt to stretch the Velcro waist band of his vest around his sizeable girth. Bryan could benefit from losing a kilogram or two and Rowdy took great pleasure in teasing him of the fact.

'I haven't put on weight,' Bryan huffed defensively, and sucked in his stomach to secure the waist band. Bryan then exhaled. The Velcro tabs began to protest when his stomach returned to its normal, bulging state. The small hooked barbs tore and ripped as they loosened their hold under the pressure, until finally becoming silent.

'There, fits perfectly,' said Bryan proudly, as he looked down at the luminous yellow vest stretched snugly around him.

'It's not that I want to insult you, Bryan,' lied Rowdy. The two officers actually took great pleasure in trading insults. 'But I think it might be a more flattering look if you leave it undone.'

'What are you, my personal stylist now?' Bryan said, and placed his police cap lopsidedly on his head to complete the ensemble.

Rowdy looked Bryan up and down, and passed a judgemental eye over his colleague. He then made another slur towards his appearance, 'Well, look at you. It's embarrassing. A sack of potatoes would look better in that uniform than you do.'

Bryan took the insult with good grace. The good natured banter had been going on between the two for years, and neither took it personally. It was a sign of the good friendship that existed between them, bonded together through many a hardship and horrific experience.

Bryan feigned a hurt look and said, 'This sack of potatoes has feelings you know.'

Rowdy could not help one last dig. 'At least potatoes have more starch in them than that shirt of yours,' he said, and pointed at the crush marks on Bryan's sleeves.

The two officers now stood at the front of the police vehicle and faced towards the oncoming traffic. One-hundred metres away, they could see Baz standing on the footpath. He had situated himself at the front of the ambulance station, dressed in his own reflective vest and cap. The majority of motorists would not even see him – it was a case of blending in by standing out. Some drivers would even assume he was an ambulance officer that posed no threat to their motoring enjoyment.

'Do you copy okay, Baz?' Rowdy asked into the handheld portable radio, on a non-operational channel. A burst of static squeaked from the radio's speaker as Rowdy released the transmit button.

'I've got you loud and clear,' Baz replied after the radio crackled at his end.

'Have you got a clear line of sight to us?' asked Rowdy, to confirm that when Baz observed a motorist not wearing a seatbelt, he could follow that same vehicle until it was stopped. The last thing they wanted was to stop the wrong car, and issue a ticket to someone who didn't deserve it. Not this time anyway.

'Yep, all's good,' Baz replied clearly.

'When you're ready then,' said Rowdy, as if raising the starter's pistol into the air and firing it off. 'Bryan's pen hand is starting to twitch.'

'Just make sure he's got plenty of ink,' Baz shot back over the airway. 'I've got a feeling were going to net a bag full.'

Rowdy walked from the front of his car, back onto the footpath. He leaned through the open front passenger door window, and retrieved an Alcolmeter from the centre console. He also grabbed a handful of the small white tubes that fitted to the top of the device. Returning beside Bryan, he stuffed the tubes into a pocket and hung the small breath testing device by its lanyard, over the grip of his sidearm.

Rowdy had never had to use his firearm in anger, and hoped he never did. 'I knew this thing would come in handy one day,' he said as he adjusted the strap of the Alcolmeter.

'Do we need to do a risk assessment for this site?' Bryan suddenly asked as the thought occurred to him.

'It's already been done,' answered Rowdy. 'It's on file back in the office.' It was only a recent introduction that written risk assessments had to be completed for police operations of any kind, in order to comply with the Occupational Health and Safety legislation.

'We're getting more like a mine site every day,' complained Bryan. 'It takes two hours to do a ten minute job, just because some idiot doesn't have the sense of self preservation.'

'It's a pity we don't get paid like a miner, though,' Rowdy added, as he considered the risks faced by a drag line operator or dump truck driver. He compared those occupations to his own, and reflected on how he was equipped with gun, capsicum spray, baton, handcuffs, and a bullet proof vest in the boot of the car.

'Someone must think we do a pretty dangerous job to give us all this equipment to protect ourselves,' Rowdy now lamented to his offsider.

'Cheer up,' Bryan laughed. 'Think of all the fun you're having.'

Formal risk assessments were still something Rowdy struggled to accept. As far as he was concerned, police had been doing risk assessments long before OH & S legislation ever existed. Today, however, it was no longer sufficient to just perform these risk assessments in your head, and adjust them by the minute as a situation changed, or escalated.

Rowdy worked on the basic concept that when you came to work, you did whatever was necessary to go home at the end of the day, and not detour via the hospital or the morgue.

A twinge struck Rowdy's back again. He winced but the short sharp pain was gone as soon as it came. 'I must have stuffed up that risk assessment of the brawl the other night,' he told Bryan as he rubbed his lower back.

The voice of Baz crackled over the radio. Rowdy and Bryan were mustered into action as the first target vehicle was called in.

Ricky had been on duty five hours, and his body was telling him it needed more fuel. His rumbling hunger pains battled for his attention over the nervous fluttering he felt, caused by the pending Internal Affairs interview.

'I'm just going to have a quick bite to eat,' he said to Tombstone, who sat surrounded by his own mountain of paperwork.

'The last meal of a condemned man,' Tombstone said flatly, and looked up from his typewriter. 'I hope it's something good?'

'Devon and tomato sauce sandwich,' replied Ricky. 'Not quite cordon bleu, but it will have to do.'

Tombstone pulled the report he was working on through the typewriter's rubber rollers. Without pushing the lever to release the tension on the rollers, the ratchet whizzed through its notches.

'I'll join you,' Tombstone said now the machine was quiet. 'Nothing worse than eating alone when you're about to face the executioner.'

'You sure know how to fill a bloke with confidence.'

Tombstone knew there was nothing he could say to Ricky which would ease his nerves. Being subjected to an Internal Affairs interview was never an enjoyable experience, regardless of your length of service.

Ricky pulled at the cling wrap surrounding his sandwich until he found a loose end. He sat opposite Tombstone in the station's meal room and forced himself to nibble away at his homemade, meagre offering, more out of physical need than desire.

'I've never asked how you got your nickname,' Ricky said to Tombstone, to make conversation and take his mind off the pending interview.

Tombstone gave one of his rare, lazy smiles and said, 'Do you remember your first day here in Chifley?'

'How could I forget it,' Ricky replied with a shocked look, as the memory of that day instantly came to him.

Tombstone's face now showed its usual stern disguise. 'Who were you working with that day?' he asked.

'As I recall, I had the pleasure of working with you that first day,' replied Ricky, just after swallowing a mouthful of sandwich.

Like most first days at any new job, Ricky spent it becoming orientated with his unfamiliar surroundings. Even though he was rostered on the truck with Tombstone that first shift, Ricky spent a good part of the day organising a place to live. The boss let him leave early in order to get the utilities, such as power, connected to the small one bedroom flat he had found to rent. Later that afternoon, however, Tombstone located Ricky and told him he had an *interesting* job for him.

Tombstone conveyed Ricky to an old, residential house, located in the heart of Chifley. On arrival, two other officers were milling around on the front lawn. Their spirits noticeably lifted when they saw Ricky, which left him in no doubt he was being set up for something. He knew it would be to his detriment and everyone else's enjoyment.

'Just go on in,' an officer said, and pointed to the open front door of the house, then chuckled lightly before his face turned to a wolfish grin.

'What do I do when I go in there?' inquired Ricky seriously.

'You'll work it out. Just follow your nose,' laughed the other officer, unable to hide his enjoyment.

Ricky warily climbed the front steps to the door. He noticed it had been forced. Splintered timber hung from the frame, the result of Tombstone having previously placed a heavy shoulder against the locked door.

Having only taken one apprehensive step inside the house, Ricky was hit with the most repulsive smell he had ever experienced. He looked back at the three officers standing in the front yard. All had a smug look as they waited with their arms crossed against their chest. One gave Ricky a wave. The other gave him a thumb up. Tombstone, just smiled inwardly.

The further inside the house Ricky moved, the stronger, and more tainted the air became. His nose led him to a bedroom. The room was dimly lit and he flicked on the light switch.

Lying in bed was the decaying remains of a once elderly woman. A bed sheet covered the lower half of her body. Her face and exposed arms were blackened from decay. The skin over her face was collapsing into the crevices of her skull as the meaty tissue beneath rotted. She would have looked right at home in the Egyptian Mummy section of any museum. The linen sheets surrounding her were stained as she slowly melted into the mattress.

It was obvious to all of Ricky's senses that the woman was dead, and had been for some time. But then, he saw her sagging cheeks move. He knew it wasn't possible, but he couldn't help but have that initial thought she was still alive.

There it was again. Both cheeks this time were definitely moving. Ricky took several tentative steps closer. The blackened lips now parted. She was trying to say something as her lips quivered. 'It's just not possible,' he repeated to himself, and moved even closer. Ricky didn't realise it, but his hand tightly gripped the handle of his sidearm.

His sense of smell had been so overwhelmed, that his other senses had no longer been as acute. It was only now that he detected a buzzing sound in the room. As his hearing came back on line, the buzzing became louder. Ricky jumped nervously when a blowfly landed on his nose and startled him. He swatted at the insect, and sent it back into the air, to swarm with the hovering black cloud that circled the ceiling.

Ricky moved to within arm's length. He raised his hand slowly and moved it towards the dead woman's neck. It just wasn't possible for her to be alive, but he felt compelled to check for a pulse. His hand was only centimetres from her face as he leaned over the bed. Ricky quickly jerked his hand away, and gasped as he saw between her parted lips.

The old lady's mouth was full of squirming maggots as they ate and burrowed their way into the soft decaying tissue of her mouth. Ricky was more relieved than horrified.

The old lady had died in her sleep four weeks previously. It was only when neighbours had not noticed her around for some time that they contacted police, and Tombstone forced his way in to discover the horrific, but sad scene.

'Poor old duck,' Ricky said to Tombstone in between chews of his sandwich as his thoughts returned to the present. 'Imagine dying alone like that, with no family to care for you.'

'You had us in stitches when you ran back out the door screaming, 'She's alive, she's alive…'' said Tombstone, without a hint of emotion.

'I couldn't let you bastard's have all the fun,' replied Ricky.

'Do you recall the night work we did together not long after that?' Tombstone asked to prompt Ricky's memory again.

Ricky didn't need time to think. 'The one with the three suicides?' he said to clarify, but knowing full well his memory was spot on. It was another of those unforgettable experiences.

'That's the one,' confirmed Tombstone.

The first four nights of this particular night roster had been relatively quiet. On the fifth night, however, Ricky and Tombstone were called to a suicide. A young man, just out of his teens, decided to end all his problems when he placed a shotgun in his mouth. He sat in the backyard of his parents' home and consumed sufficient alcohol to actually pull the trigger. His head exploded.

On the sixth night, Tombstone took the call from a person who had heard a gunshot in a neighbouring house. Ricky and Tombstone arrived to find another young man had placed a .22 calibre magnum in his mouth. He pulled the trigger while sitting on the bathroom floor.

On this occasion, though, the young man was the son of one of the local court staff. The smaller calibre rifle caused much less physical disfigurement than the shot gun, but the result was the same. They found the young man lying in a pool of congealing blood. After completing their investigation and the body snatchers had removed the corpse, Ricky and Tombstone cleaned the bathroom, and washed litres of blood down the floor sump. The last thing Tombstone had wanted was for the boy's mother to be left with the sickening aftermath.

'You're a very thoughtful bloke, Tombstone.'

If the compliment caused the veteran officer to be embarrassed, he failed to show it. Ricky did not see the dark cloud that passed across Tombstone's eyes.

'You do what's right,' Tombstone replied.

The seventh and final night started with another suicide. It occurred on a remote property, thirty kilometres from town. A desperate farmer did the only thing he felt he could do to escape his circumstances. He placed a .22 calibre rifle under his chin and pulled the trigger. The result was ultimately the same as the previous two suicides, but initially more confronting. Ricky and Tombstone arrived at the property before the ambulance, and were confronted with the farmer, who should have been dead, but was still alive. He lay on the ground unconscious. The man's chest still heaved with each strained breath as his respiratory system refused to shut down. Blood gurgled, as it frothed from his mouth and nose. He moaned loudly, not so much from pain that raked his subconscious but as his body's final protest against its fate, which would later come in an ambulance on route to hospital.

Ricky remembered the shock he felt as he stood above the dying man. His shock then turned to utter helplessness as family members screamed and begged him to help their dying husband and father.

'I don't ever want to feel like that again,' said Ricky with his head lowered, as he fought back the emotion that threatened.

Tombstone could hear the remorse in Ricky's voice and rose from the meal table. He headed for the sink, giving the young officer space to gather his emotions.

'It was certainly a night work to remember,' Tombstone said with his back turned, and rinsed his plate. 'Do you remember the next dead'n after that?'

Ricky paused a moment to clear his mind of the farmer's dying image before answering. 'It was that guy on the train line,' he finally said. His head filled with a fresh volley of disturbing images.

'Who were you working with?' asked Tombstone.

'You, again,' replied Ricky.

On this occasion, Ricky and Tombstone were called to the rail line, a few hundred metres south of Chifley Train Station. On arrival, they discovered the aftermath of another suicide. A young man decided to end his life by walking into the path of a freight train travelling at speed. Needless to say, he came off second best. His body exploded. Every limb was torn away from the man's torso which was then reduced to pulp. Internal organs were scattered across the surrounding field in a fifty metre arc. The recovery process of the body parts in the long grass was arduous. Most often, organs were only located when something soft was felt under foot. In the end, they recovered enough of the man to pose a serious jigsaw puzzle challenge for the pathologist.

'At least one good thing came out of it,' Tombstone joked as they discussed the incident. 'He made the post mortem easy for the doctor.'

Ricky had been trying to force himself to eat his sandwich, but most still lay on the cling-wrap in front of him. He had not had much of an appetite but he had even less now after the morbid table talk.

'I think I see why you got the nickname, Tombstone,' said Ricky, as he wrapped his sandwich to toss into the garbage.

'And they are just some of the dead'ns we've done together,' said Tombstone as he sat back at the meal table. 'Not to mention all the others I've done over the years.'

'At least we've got our dead'n over and done with today,' Ricky tried to bolster his spirits.

'This would be a good time to mention then that I have done more than one per shift.'

'That's okay,' replied Ricky and checked the time on his wrist watch. 'You might be looking for a new partner if this IA interview doesn't go well.'

Dick walked up to the pretty blonde receptionist at Kingstown Morgue. 'Good morning,' he greeted cheerfully.

The entrance and reception area of the morgue was brightly lit and tastefully decorated. It would not have been out of place in any modern commercial office complex. The walls were painted in vibrant colours and were lined with numerous seascapes of the nearby coastline. Dick had never thought much about what the reception area to a morgue should look like, but these crisp surroundings always surprised him when he entered. It certainly gave no clues to what lay on the other side of the wall.

'Good morning, sir,' replied the receptionist through perfectly aligned white teeth. 'How can I help you today?'

'I'm here to see one of your clients,' said Dick with an attempt at humour. If the receptionist found his comment even remotely funny, she failed to show it. Her lips covered the white teeth and her pleasant smile vanished, replaced with a look of confusion.

Dick took a more serious approach this time to help the young girl out. 'I'm here to fingerprint a drowning victim brought in from the Benstown area.'

The receptionist did not say a word as she started to tap away at her computer keyboard. Her smile returned. 'That will be number 1509/06,' she said, and efficiently wrote the number onto an admission card, which she then placed on the counter top in front of Dick. It was soon followed by a locker key.

'Please fill in our admission book with the card details and locker key number,' she continued, with another smile and flash of pearly whites. Dick realised the pleasant smile that spread across the girl's face after saying anything was just done out of habit and masked politeness.

'I'd love to,' Dick said sarcastically with his own false smile.

Dick commenced the entry in the admission book on the counter top. As he wrote, he heard the receptionist take several deep sniffs that caused her nostrils to flare.

Dick could not help himself as he realised his clothing still wafted. 'Don't worry, it's not you. That pleasant odour is my new aftershave. Do you like it?' The receptionist did not reply, either out of politeness or ignorance, Dick couldn't tell which. She just smiled again.

'Just go through that door,' she pointed. 'You'll find a locker to secure your gun and then give the admission card to the attendant,' she said, and again finished with a cheesy grin.

Third time lucky, Dick thought to himself as he again made an attempt at humour to achieve some sort of human interaction with the girl. 'But I may need my gun,' he said seriously to the smiling face, only to watch it again instantly vanish. 'What happens if one of your client's moves or tries to get off the table? I have to be able to defend myself.'

Again, an awkward silence greeted Dick until the receptionist finally replied, 'Department of Health policy. No firearms allowed,' and smiled.

Dick had to admit defeat. It was time to try a new audience. Perhaps the ones lying in cold storage, on the other side of the door, would have more personality than the pretty young blonde receptionist.

12.30PM

Baz had been keeping Rowdy and Bryan busy over the last half hour. No sooner had they stopped and dealt with one traffic offender, the voice of Baz would crackle from the portable radio with another to be stopped.

Most of the drivers stopped accepted their fate. Some did not realise they had forgotten to put on their seatbelts and were genuinely shocked by the oversight. Most were apologetic and promised never to do it again in a bid to avoid a fine. Some women would become tearful in their attempts to avoid the consequences, while others were genuinely upset by their first encounter with police.

Rowdy and Bryan had both been around long enough to know which response was which, neither could be seduced by fluttering eyelids. Rowdy considered himself a good judge of character, and whether a person was being authentic in their response.

Half of the motorists Rowdy stopped in the last half hour received a caution. He would still record their details in his notebook, but no ticket would be issued. He was sensible enough to know, however, that his judgement was not perfect, and there would always be a percentage of drivers who were good actors, or cons, and would put one over him. Rowdy accepted this was the price he had to pay for performing his role with compassion. Although his memory for names might not have been the best, he never forgot a face. One of the most truly satisfying times that Rowdy's job provided, was when he re-encountered one of those faces that had conned him.

Bryan approached the role differently. He lived by the motto, *In God we trust. Everyone else is a suspect.*

He showed little leniency and felt the fairest way to perform his role was to give everyone a ticket.

Bryan finished issuing another fine and sent the driver on his way. He walked back towards Rowdy, retrieved a handkerchief from a trouser pocket and wiped the sweat at the back of his neck. Dark sweat stains had appeared under his arms, and his shirt tail had managed to untuck itself, hanging shabbily over his gun belt.

In contrast, Rowdy's appearance was still as immaculate as when he had commenced his shift. He lazed back, resting his backside on the bonnet of the police vehicle. He tilted his head skyward and closed his eyes under the peak of his cap, and let his mind relax. He felt the warm sun tingle his face, which was the only exposed part of his body. His skin was susceptible to skin cancers, so he always wore long sleeved shirts.

Rowdy felt the suns intensity strengthen, and the tingling sensation became warmth that penetrated deep into the pores of his skin. The spreading warmth quickly started to burn, as the sun's full intensity threatened to sear deep into his skin. He felt his eyes begin to warm as the sun pierced through the thin skin of his eyelids.

It was one of those rare occasions that Rowdy was immersed in the moment. No thoughts of the past were shown as replays in his mind. The seatbelt enforcement melted away with the sun's rays. Any anxiety of what the future may hold vanished, as the sounds, and smell of passing traffic, only a metre away, was exchanged for the yodelling song of a magpie perched in the tree above him. He could even smell the freshly mowed grass in the park.

'Red commodore sedan. Bravo Romeo Yankee Five Seven Two. Driver only occupant,' came the voice from the radio. Rowdy lowered his head before opening his eyes. At the same time he pushed off the bonnet of his car, turned and faced the oncoming traffic.

He spotted the target vehicle and saw the driver was wearing a plain red T-shirt to match the colour of his car. Rowdy looked for the black strap of the seatbelt crossing the man's chest, but found none. The seatbelt buckle was still hanging beside the driver's right shoulder, clearly visible as the sun reflected off it. Rowdy would make a note of all these details on the police copy of the ticket, if he issued one.

Rowdy stepped partially into the path of the approaching vehicle and pointed directly at the driver. He then signalled him to pull into the kerb, in front of the police vehicle. The driver still made no reaction to put on his seatbelt as many before him had.

'Correct vehicle,' the voice confirmed from the radio.

Rowdy walked slowly up to the driver's door, peering through the rear window of the car as he approached. It was a routine that was second nature to Rowdy. A quick look to check if there was anything, or anybody secreted in the back that may pose a threat. After all, Rowdy had no idea who he was stopping. It could be anyone, from the average Joe, to an armed robber, or a drug supplier.

'Good afternoon, sir,' said Rowdy cheerfully. He stood just behind the driver. The driver had to twist his body, and turn his head, placing him off balance in order to see Rowdy.

'You have been observed not wearing your seatbelt. May I please see your driver's licence?'

'Do you think you're being funny or something?' came the driver's unexpected response.

'No sir,' said Rowdy, somewhat confused. 'I take seatbelt offences seriously.' Rowdy's mind raced as he tried to work out the angle the man was trying to use to get out of this fine.

'Are you having a go at me?' he said, adding to Rowdy's confusion.

'I can assure you, sir, that the only reason we are standing here talking is because you were observed not wearing your seatbelt.'

The conversation kept getting more bizarre when the driver asked in a more aggressive tone. 'Why do you have to insult me on that sign?'

'Sir, I have no idea what you are talking about,' Rowdy said in total bewilderment. He now assumed he had a real crackpot on his hands.

'The sign you've got flashing,' continued the driver, and pointed backwards with his thumb out the window. 'I personally find that offensive.'

'What... the light-bar?' exclaimed Rowdy, still trying to make sense of the conversation.

The only sign that Rowdy could assume the driver was referring to was the *Buckle Up* message scrolling across the police vehicle's roof mounted message bar.

'I want your name and station,' the driver continued to rant. 'You're not going to get away with this. You can't 'Up Bickle' me.'

Rowdy had no idea what the driver was going on about. He knew better than to try and be rational with an irrational person and gave up on any further conversation to make sense of the situation.

'Show me your licence, sir,' Rowdy demanded.

The driver cursed incoherently as he struggled to remove his wallet from a rear pocket of his trousers. Spittle shot from his mouth as he continued to rave, with only every fourth or fifth word discernible.

'........sacked...........job............ombudsman.........arsehole.'

The driver's arm shot aggressively out the window as he produced his driver's licence. Rowdy checked the expiry date and read the name, 'Ronald John Bickle.' The penny finally dropped, as Rowdy pieced the conversation together.

'I won't keep you long, sir,' said Rowdy and turned away, stifling a laugh.

Rowdy picked up his ticket book off the bonnet of the highway car, and then checked the message bar. Sure enough, 'Buckle Up' was still scrolling across.

'That bloke doesn't sound too happy,' said Bryan, as Rowdy returned to the front of the highway car.

'He thinks our message bar is scrolling 'Up Bickle,' explained Rowdy, and handed across the driver's licence for Bryan to read.

Bryan started to laugh as he read the name. 'You're not serious?'

'He is apparently,' Rowdy chuckled, and took the licence back. 'So serious in fact, he's going to get me fired over it.'

'And rightly so,' said Bryan critically. 'You can't go around personally insulting everyone you stop like that.'

Rowdy finished writing out the infringement notice. 'This should be interesting,' he said as he removed the completed ticket, and walked back to the driver's door.

Handing over the driver's licence first, Rowdy then said, 'Sir, this is an infringement notice for the offence of not wearing a seatbelt. Its full method of disposal is explained on the back.' Rowdy disregarded the idea of trying to explain to the confused driver his misunderstanding about the sign.

'You will also see on the back I've written my name, and station for you, along with a contact phone number for the police station,' said Rowdy helpfully.

The driver snatched the ticket from Rowdy's hand, scrunched it into a ball and threw it onto the floor of the car. 'Is there any particular reason why you weren't wearing a seatbelt?'

'I never wear it,' the driver snapped. 'More people have been killed by wearing a seatbelt than not.'

Rowdy smiled and made no attempt to hide his enjoyment when he said, 'Well, if you choose not to put it on when you drive away from here, then I will happily post you out another infringement.'

'You won't get away with this,' the driver said as he buckled up his seatbelt, and then accelerated.

'Have a safe journey,' Rowdy said to the departing car as he turned to stroll back to Bryan. 'Why do I get all the nutters?' he said to Bryan with a shake of his head. '… and you always get the good looking ones.'

Dick dutifully secured his firearm into a locker and pocketed the key. 'Won't be a minute, mate,' a morgue assistant called out, as he passed through the admission area.

The morgue assistant was dressed in white from head to toe. He would have looked right at home in any hospital operating theatre. Dick watched through a glass panel as the assistant grabbed a handheld shower nozzle from the tiled wall. Water jetted from the nozzle as he held it towards himself, and washed down the white plastic apron that covered him down to his gum boots. The blood covering the apron faded as it was diluted by the water, and streamed like a waterfall from the bottom of the apron, until it swirled around, to finally disappear down a floor drain.

Dick could not help but think that a person had to be just a little odd to work in this place. After all, how could you wake up every morning and look forward to coming to this. Then again, some people may think the very same of Dick's job.

'Sorry to keep you,' the morgue assistant said happily as he approached, still wiping off excess water from his apron with a towel. 'What can I do for you?'

'I'm here to fingerprint 1509/06,' Dick said, and handed over the admission card.

'Ah, the drowning victim,' the assistant replied, recognising the number. 'I can't wait until we get rid of that one,' he continued.

Dick did not need any explanation though. He could already imagine the sight of the bloated, half eaten body, and smell the putrid flesh. 'Come on through,' gestured the assistant. 'Just grab your protective clothing off the shelves.'

Dick started to dress himself from the selection of light blue clothing on offer. He placed a hair net over his head. At first he stretched it too far and covered his eyes, but quickly pulled the front up. He donned a surgical gown, and like most men, fumbled to secure the ties behind his back. Dick sat on a wall mounted bench-seat, and slipped on a pair of waterproof, protective shoe covers with non-slip soles. He rose back to his feet before glancing at his reflection in a glass panelled wall, and checked his gown was hanging right. He grabbed a pair of safety glasses and dust mask off the shelving to complete the outfit.

No matter how clean the morgue looked with its tiles shimmering under the harsh fluorescent lighting, Dick just accepted he was in a dirty place, and was not fooled by the shiny surroundings. He would try to avoid coming into unnecessary contact with any surface. Until he left the premises, and had scrubbed the skin from his hands, at no stage would he touch his face, or any other part of his body. As usual, the minute Dick reminded himself of this, every part of his face and body would scream out to be scratched.

The protective clothing was also necessary to avoid any contamination of the deceased by the pathologist, morgue attendants, or in this case, the police.

The morgue assistant led Dick past a series of rooms which were used as viewing, or counselling rooms for relatives of the deceased.

Grief counsellors could also be on hand to assist relatives when they were called upon to identify their loved one.

The person's death alone was reason enough for the family to be distressed. Adding the need for an autopsy caused many to become distraught. It requires delicate handling by trained professionals to explain the necessity of a post mortem. Apart from the judicial requirements to establish the cause of a death, whether by natural or criminal means, there is also an educational and public health aspect to the procedure. The autopsy may provide family members with information about diseases, which may prevent their own premature death. 'Are you busy at the moment,' Dick asked the morgue assistant, making conversation.'

'Yeah, we've got a full house,' the assistant replied casually. 'You know how it is; people are just dying to stay here.'

Finally, someone with a sense of humour, Dick thought. 'And I thought my jokes were bad,' Dick remarked with a chuckle. 'It's not quite what I would consider tropical resort weather you have in here,' Dick continued as the drop in temperature caused a chilly shudder through his body.

'You'll get used to it,' replied the assistant maintaining his humour.

'I hope not,' Dick said. 'I don't plan on staying that long.'

'It's only cold enough to preserve the bodies, not freeze them,' explained the morgue assistant. 'It's just a big cool room really.'

Dick knew he was approaching the main cool room where all the bodies were stored, and he noticed a definite change in odour that permeated the cool moist air. Just what he needed, an even fouler stench impregnated into his clothing than he already had.

'Doesn't the smell get to you?' asked Dick.

The morgue assistant turned his head over a shoulder to face Dick while still walking. An amused expression spread over his face by the question everyone who enters his work place asked him. 'What smell?' he replied with a silly grin. His olfactory had long become accustomed to its surroundings.

The morgue assistant pushed through a set of double swing doors, into the main cool room. The large storage room was completely full of stainless steel trolleys, with only enough space for a person to walk between. Each trolley had a zippered bag on top, with its own unique identification label attached. Even with the exhaust fans running, the smell was intense. The coldness prevented the bodies from decaying any further, but it did nothing to suppress the unique smell of those bodies which had already started to rot, prior to being delivered. It was not a gut wrenching smell so much as just being unpleasant. But it was a smell that permeated into every pore of your skin. For hours after leaving the morgue, Dick would still be reminded of its odour as the lining of his nose and nasal hairs were painted with it. Had it not been for the surroundings, the smell was probably no different to walking into any butcher's shop.

Dick was amazed at the number of bodies stored in the room. It did not resemble the storage rooms portrayed in American movies. There were no banks of individual storage fridges, lining the walls from floor to ceiling, from which a body would be effortlessly rolled out.

'You need a multilevel car park,' Dick joked at the congestion.

'Just goes to show how busy we are,' said the assistant. 'We have a pretty quick turnaround. Most autopsies are done within twenty-four hours of landing here, and then return to the funeral directors.'

'It really is a meat factory,' Dick said in wonderment, more to himself than to the assistant, as he looked across row after row of bodies.

'I hope my bloke is near the front?' asked Dick, as he was contemplating how they were going to get a trolley out from the middle of the room.

'Actually, the autopsy has already been done on your bloke,' the morgue assistant said, as he pushed his way through another set of double swing doors on the opposite side of the room. 'We've got him ready for you in here.'

Dick followed the assistant through the doors. Even though he knew he was entering the main surgical room, he was always brought up short when confronted with it. Today was no different. Dick paused momentarily after entering, his eyes darting from one stainless steel surgical table to another. There were four in total. Each table was currently in use, with what could once be described as four bodies, lying prone upon the table's icy surface. All the bodies were in various stages of post mortem. One table was different to the others. It had a stainless steel bucket sitting at one end, near the feet of the table's occupant.

'Sorry, we can't give you a separate work area at the moment,' said the morgue assistant sincerely, while standing next to the bucket with a hand placed on its rim. 'But your bloke is in here.'

A frown was fixed on Ricky's face as he sat nervously in the interview room of Chifley Police Station, drumming his fingers on the armrest of his chair. He swivelled the creaking chair from side to side, and studied the paint peeling from the walls. The room was devoid of anything that may bring pleasure to the eye. The centre of the room housed a battered and chipped timber topped desk, supported on a black tubular frame.

The only item to decorate the desk was a typewriter. Several chairs, that looked like they had just come from the second hand shop, with their stained and torn upholstery, faced either side of the table.

The only other fixture in the room was the dual florescent light that hung precariously on chains from the ceiling.

The room's lack of decor fitted perfectly with Ricky's sombre mood, as he sat contemplating what was in store for him. His stomach still fluttered with nerves.

Ricky's thoughts then turned to the countless other poor souls who had sat in this same room, feeling the same as he. How many had been innocent, just like Ricky, and had to rely on the rules of law to protect that innocence. At least one good thing would come out of this process, he thought, as he tried to cheer himself up. He would be more aware in the future, when he was the one sitting on the other side of the desk asking the questions, instead of answering them, the importance of carrying out a thorough and ethical investigation.

Ricky sprang from his chair and stood at attention as the Internal Affairs inspector, followed by a sergeant, entered.

'Relax son,' the inspector said, as he held out his hand to shake. 'We haven't brought the firing squad today.'

Ricky took the inspector's hand firmly, and then noticed how sweaty his own palm was.

'I'm Inspector Bilson,' he said, wiping his hand on a trouser leg after releasing Ricky's hand. 'And this is Sergeant Wostic.'

'Good to meet you,' Ricky replied and relaxed somewhat as he shook the sergeant's hand.

'Please, sit down,' motioned the inspector.

'Thank you, sir,' Ricky said politely, and resumed his seat.

'I see that academy discipline hasn't left you yet,' the inspector said with an appreciative grin.

'I think my parents should get more of the credit than the academy, sir,' replied Ricky.

The Internal Affairs sergeant took a seat behind the typewriter, removed a blank piece of paper from his folder that he had placed on the desk.

He fed the paper into the machine and immediately started to type the heading details for the Record of Interview that was to follow.

Ricky watched the inspector as he took a relaxed pose in the chair beside his sergeant. Rather than rest his open folder on the desk in front of him, the inspector lay back slightly in the chair, crossed a leg over one knee, and rested the folder in his lap. Although the civil introductions had made Ricky feel more at ease, he was still alert, and was not going to be drawn into a false sense of security, or friendliness. As far as he was concerned, the two senior police officers sitting opposite were far from being colleagues. They were the enemy, and not to be trusted.

'Now, as you have already been informed, we are investigating a complaint by one…' The inspector paused to refer to his open folder, 'One Simon Dean Baker. Mr. Baker is alleging that he was assaulted when arrested by you and Senior Constable Henry Wentworth.'

'Yes, Sir,' Ricky replied, but then quickly added, to avoid any confusion from his reply. 'I mean, yes, I'm aware of that complaint.' Good one idiot, Ricky thought to himself. Nothing like confessing before the interview even starts.

'I want you to understand that this Record of Interview is subject to the same rules of evidence as any other criminal investigation. You will be given the same caution and adoption questions as any statement would be. Do you understand that?' the Inspector said, with an air of authority that made Ricky tense once more.

'Yes, sir,' said Ricky, staring directly at the inspector.

'Ready, sergeant?' he inquired of his partner.

'Ready,' his short reply came, followed by the frantic tapping of keys as he typed the official caution which gave Ricky the right not to answer any questions.

As the Inspector spoke, the sergeant typed the conversation, word for word.

'This is a copy of the duty roster for the fifth of February,' said the Inspector, passing the document across the table to Ricky. 'Do you agree that you were rostered on from three until eleven-thirty that night, as driver of Chifley 10?'

'Yes, sir,' Ricky answered, after verifying the document.

The Inspector produced the motor vehicle diary entry that Ricky had made for that shift, along with charge records of the offender. Ricky confirmed the correctness of all the documents.

'Can you now tell me what led to the arrest of Mr. Baker?' asked the Inspector. The Sergeant typed, not missing a word.

'It was about ten when I was driving up Rocket Street. Henry and I were going to do one last patrol of that area before returning to the station. The previous week had seen a number of break and enters in the area,' Ricky answered in some detail, wanting to give an accurate account of the event. 'Whilst in Rocket Street, Henry and I observed a person walking along the footpath, in the same direction as we were travelling.'

'So this person had his back to you?' the Inspector clarified.

'That's right,' replied Ricky. 'The offender then…' Ricky was cut off when the Inspector interrupted.

'Did you know he was an offender at that time?'

'No,' Ricky answered. 'We didn't know who he was then.'

'So what prompted your suspicion towards this *unknown person*? the Inspector inquired.

Ricky could now remember the incident vividly, and did not have to hesitate in his answer. 'He looked over his shoulder, back towards us. I'm assuming he heard the police truck rattling up the road. He started to run flat out along the footpath, away from us.'

'How far away from him were you when this happened?' asked the Inspector.

'About fifty metres,' Ricky recalled.

'Senior Constable Wentworth say anything to you at the time?'

Ricky did not respond immediately. He closed his eyes briefly to place himself back inside the police truck eight months ago. 'It was something similar to, 'Get up there," he finally replied.

'What happened then?'

'I accelerated as quickly as the truck could, caught up to the offender just as he ran into some dense bushes of a small nature reserve at the top end of the street,' replied Ricky confidently.

'I'll just hold you up there,' the Sergeant interjected. 'I need to make another page change.' The Sergeant fed another sheet of paper into the typewriter and completed the continuation heading.

1PM

'What happened when Mr. Baker ran into the bushes?' the Internal Affairs Inspector asked Ricky.

'I mounted the kerb and stopped the police truck about two metres short of the bushes. Senior Constable Wentworth was out of the truck before it fully stopped and ran into the bushes behind the offender.'

'Did Senior Constable Wentworth take a baton with him?' asked the Inspector pointedly.

Ricky paused before answering as he gave the question serious thought. 'No, I don't believe he did,' replied Ricky honestly.

Ricky could recall clearly that Henry had not taken a baton out of the vehicle when he chased after the offender. He did recall, however, that he grabbed one of the Maglite torches before giving chase. Ricky only answered the question asked and did not volunteer any additional information.

'Were the headlights of your vehicle directed into the bushes?' asked the Inspector, making it clear what he was alluding to.

'Yes, they were,' replied Ricky, and anticipated what the next question would be.

Ricky's assumption was correct when the Inspector asked, 'Could you see Mr. Baker or Senior Constable Wentworth once they entered the bushes?'

'No, not at all,' came Ricky's immediate reply.

'What happened then?' prompted the Inspector.

'By the time I stopped and parked the vehicle, they had both disappeared into the bushes. I approached and was about to enter the shrubbery when I heard the rustle of bushes, followed by an agonising groan.'

'Could you recognise whose voice it was?' the Inspector queried.

'No, I couldn't,' replied Ricky.

'And then?' the Inspector cued Ricky on.

'I recall I hesitated slightly. I considered returning to the police truck to call for backup, and to alert the station of our location, before entering the bushes,' explained Ricky.

'And did you?' asked the Inspector with some curiosity.

'No, I entered the bushes calling out to Henry, asking if he was okay,' Ricky responded.

'Did Senior Constable Wentworth answer you back?' probed the Inspector.

'Yes. He said he was alright and then I met up with him a few metres into the bushes. He was escorting the offender out,' answered Ricky.

'Did Senior Constable Wentworth say anything else?'

'Yes, he said the offender tripped over a tree root, and I saw that he was bleeding slightly from the head,' replied Ricky.

'Did Mr. Baker say anything at this time,' the Inspector asked, continuing to explore into the event.

'No, nothing,' said Ricky. 'We searched him and found the cash and jewellery in his pockets, and questioned him about that. At no stage did he complain or say anything about the small cut on his head the whole time he was in our custody,' said Ricky, to make it perfectly clear that there was no complaint of assault from the offender at the time.

'Mr. Baker claims that one of you struck him on the head with a baton,' the Inspector stated and waited for a reply.

Ricky was again pleased that the question specified a baton and he could answer honestly, 'At no stage did Senior Constable Wentworth, or I, remove our batons from the vehicle,' he responded with confidence.

Ricky was thankful that he did not witness how the offender sustained the injury. While he had no reason to doubt what Henry had said to him, he knew that there was the possibility that the torch Henry carried into the bushes, may have carelessly slipped out of his hand in the struggle to apprehend the thief, and by some unfortunate act of fate, come into contact with the thief's head.

'Is there anything else you wish to add?' asked the Inspector.

'No, nothing at all,' Ricky said as he now sat comfortably in his chair for the first time.

The Sergeant typed the adoption questions which Ricky answered, and then signed each page of the record of interview. To the Sergeant's credit, there were only two typos that required initialling.

'Well done son,' the Internal Affairs Inspector said as he rose from his chair, having collated his folder back into order. Ricky rose with him and again shook the hand that was offered. He noticed that the Inspector did not have to wipe his hand on his trousers this time.

'You answered the specific questions well,' the Inspector said with a knowing look, which said more than the words spoken.

'What happens now?' asked Ricky.

'We still have to interview Senior Constable Wentworth, but I foresee no problems there. It's obviously a malicious complaint has been made by a revengeful offender that has no basis of truth whatsoever,' the Inspector said cheerfully.

Internal Affairs are not that bad after all, Ricky thought to himself as he left the room and headed back to the front station area.

'Pass me your phone, please hon,' Lynda Crisp said to her husband while she fossicked through her handbag cradled in her lap.

'What are you looking for?' Lindsay replied, and stretched back in his car seat to try and retrieve his mobile phone from a trouser pocket.

'I wrote the phone number down of the airport on a piece of paper. It's in here somewhere,' Lynda explained, as she now started to remove the contents of her handbag, one by one.

Lindsay just shook his head as the collection of odds and ends that comprise a woman's handbag were revealed. There were enough Band-Aids to secure a severed leg, and then paracetamol tablets to subdue the pain. If you happened to come into contact with poison ivy, just before severing your leg, then there was a blister pack of antihistamine, and a tube of cream that vowed to cure every ailment known to modern medicine. More blister packs were removed, this time to treat both constipation and diarrhoea, as if the severed leg and itching were not bad enough. A small bottle of waterless antibacterial hand sanitiser appeared and was added to the growing pile, along with four different types of throat lozenges. The bag was half empty when the hair brush and cosmetic items started to appear, along with sanitary pads, and four nail files just in case you broke the other three.

'You've got more stock in there than the local chemist,' Lindsay said in amazement as he passed his mobile phone across.

'You never know when you'll need something,' Lynda replied without looking up from her endeavour. 'Remember that time we climbed to the top of Mount Kosciusko, and there was that poor woman with all those blisters on her feet. Who was able to treat her and get her back down from the summit?'

'You dear,' Lindsay replied, followed by an affectionate pat to his wife's arm.

'That's right and… ahhh, got it,' she said triumphantly as she removed a crumpled piece of paper and started to smooth it out.

Lynda quickly repacked her handbag and then dialled the airport number to confirm if her son's flight was running on time.

'What did they say?' Lindsay inquired as his wife disconnected the call and placed the mobile phone into the console between the seats.

'At the moment the flight is on schedule, so we should arrive with time to spare,' replied Lynda, checking her watch.

The couple had just entered one of the many small rural towns they would pass through on their journey to Sydney.

'Why don't we stop for some lunch at that bakery,' said Lynda as she pointed towards a large sign mounted on the front awning of a shop.

'I could go for a nice warm pie,' Lindsay said. He could already smell the warm pastry treat as he imagined himself biting into 'Grandma's Best Pie', or so the advertising sign claimed. The fantasy was short lived.

'No you won't,' Lynda said adamantly. 'You know what the doctor said about your cholesterol. You'll have a nice fresh salad sandwich.'

'Just one won't hurt,' Lindsay pleaded his lost cause. 'After all, it's a special day, picking the boy up and all.'

'Meat pies will kill you,' Lynda stated.

'I guess a nice caramel tart for dessert is out of the question then?' Lindsay said just to stir his wife as he parked the car in front of the bakery.

Lindsay grabbed his phone as he got out of the car, and placed it back into his trouser pocket. He took his wife's hand as they had done since teenagers, and walked the short distance to the bakery for a healthy lunch.

Dick peered into the bucket which was half filled with water. Partly submerged, were two grotesque hands which had been severed at the wrist joint.

'The rest of the body absolutely reeks,' said the morgue assistant. 'We left it under wraps to avoid smelling the whole place out again. We removed the hands to make it more pleasant for you.'

'I appreciate that,' Dick said vacantly as he starred into the bucket.

'If you need anything, just let me know,' offered the morgue assistant as he walked over to one of the other tables.

'I should be fine,' said Dick, and could not help the next wisecrack. 'I've got an extra hand here already.'

'And you had the hide to complain about my jokes,' the assistant laughed as he settled a clear, protective face shield on his head, then flipped down its clear visor and started to remove the rib cage from a corpse.

Dick's eyes managed to slowly move their gaze away from the floating hands to the feet, that were resting against the bucket. He raised his head to follow the hairy limbs all the way up to the genitals of the naked corpse, which confirmed his suspicions that the legs belonged to a male. From the groin up though, all resemblance of a once living human-being, vanished.

A large incision had been made across the man's chest from shoulder to shoulder, and then down the length of the torso to the pubic bone. The skin, and soft meaty tissue just under its surface, had been peeled back to reveal the rib cage. The top flap was pulled up to partly cover the face and expose the neck muscles. The rib cage had then been removed to expose the internal organs. Various cuts had then been made to arteries and ligaments. Any attachment to the spinal cord, bladder, and then rectum had been severed, in order to remove the internal organs in one piece. The organs were then placed aside for further examination and weighing. Tissue samples would be taken if required and the major blood vessels examined. Even the contents of the stomach would be examined, which can contribute to determine the time of death.

'That's one way to lose weight,' said Dick to himself as he looked into the empty cave of the man's torso.

The skin covering the head had been cut from ear to ear. The front portion of the scalp had been pulled away from the skull and draped over the face. The rear flap had been pulled back over the neck. The top of the exposed skull had been cut and removed to expose the brain, which was now sitting on the steel table beside the head.

Dick looked across to the table beside him. Another morgue assistant worked methodically to restore a body back to its former glory after having had the autopsy completed. He was sewing the skull flaps back together to retain the 'skull cap' that had previously been removed. He would then dump the internal organs, which were now secure inside a bright yellow plastic bag, back into the exposed cavity before suturing the chest flaps back together with the dexterity of a seamstress.

Dick could not help but imagine the archaeologists in years to come, digging up long forgotten grave sites and finding these plastic bags along with the skeletal remains. What strange and marvellous burial rituals would they deduce had occurred? Just as we today try to make sense of a medieval or bronze age entombment.

Dick placed on a pair of latex surgical gloves and was just about to move the lower legs of the corpse when he stopped and said quietly, 'Just to be sure.' He then grabbed another pair of gloves and feed them onto his hands over the first. Giving the cuffs a satisfactory snap, he then delicately pushed the legs to one side and said, 'Sorry mate, but I need to use some more of your bed.'

The autopsy room was far from being a solemn place.

It was full of chatter and laughter as the medical pathologists and assistants went about their work. It was the same social chatter that went on in any workplace. Nights out were organised and sporting events were dissected with the same expert knowledge that all armchair observers possess. Although the bodies that lay before them had been impersonalised, Dick felt no shock, at what an outsider may see to be disrespectful or inappropriate. He knew full well that this social banter was a necessary coping mechanism for them all.

Detachment from the individual that lay on the table was paramount. No person could survive the emotional roller coaster that accompanies death without that detachment, when faced on a daily basis.

That same detachment causes its own series of problems, which in Dick's case, had been festering below the surface for many years.

As Dick looked about the room and at the horror that was on display, he felt an overwhelming calmness slowly drape over his body. He knew death did not have to be represented by these dismembered bodies that surrounded him. He had experienced death first hand when his mother had died. All her life, she had nurtured and taught Dick all the skills he needed to live a healthy and fulfilled life. And so she continued that teaching, with her final lesson in death.

Dick had watched as she lay in a hospital bed, her body ravaged with cancer. He watched in total awe at how peaceful and beautiful an experience it was to see her take that last, long breath, and exhale for the very last time. In that moment, he knew that his mother was the victor in life and not the cancer in death. He watched as his mother met her God and triumphed over death. The tears and grief that quickly followed were not for his mother's passing. They were for his selfish feelings of loss.

'OK, time to get acquainted,' Dick said to the hands as he reached into the bucket and took hold of one.

'Pleased to meet you,' he continued to say as he shook the hand and removed some of the excess water.

Dick reached into the bucket for a second time and removed the other hand. He placed it on the cold, stainless steel table beside the first. Both hands had their palms facing upwards.

'Well that looks odd,' he said as he straightened, and took a half step backwards, while at the same time tilting his head to one side. Something was not right. Then Dick realised what the problem was; the strange thing was not that he had two severed hands lying before him, it was the fact that their thumbs were facing inwards to each other. They looked deformed.

Dick could not help himself. Just like a card shark's sleight of hand, he took the two hands and rotated their position on the table.

'That's better,' Dick said with a nod of his head, satisfied with the hands positioned with their thumbs in the outward position.

'Are you right there, mate?' the morgue assistant at the adjacent table enquired.

'I am now,' Dick replied.

'You'll let me know if they start talking back to you,' said the assistant, grinning.

'I knew I should have kept my gun.'

Baz kept Rowdy and Bryan busy with a steady stream of seatbelt offenders. Rowdy had just finished dealing with a young couple and their two children, who were heading away on holidays. As their vehicle passed, Baz noticed one of the children turned around on the rear seat to look out the back window. He called the vehicle and unrestrained child through to Rowdy.

The parents were shocked when Rowdy pointed out to them that their five-year old was not wearing a seatbelt.

He was disappointed to hear the mother say to the child, 'Tommy, put your seatbelt on or the policeman will lock you up.' The happy and inquisitive face of the five-year old turned to fear as he rushed to put his seatbelt on and then lowered his head, from both fright and shame.

Rowdy hated how parents taught their children to fear police. Seeing a perfect opportunity to reverse the situation, he spent considerable time talking with the family and eventually won over the trust of little Tommy and the other child. Letting them get into the police car to turn on the lights and sirens did the trick.

It turned out that Tommy had actually spotted Baz standing on the footpath, and was so excited to see a real live policeman that he had unbuckled himself and turned around to watch. As it was Baz' fault that the whole incident happened, Rowdy let the couple off with a caution. It was the best twenty minutes work he had done today.

Baz called in the next vehicle and as Rowdy walked out onto the roadway to signal the driver to stop, he clearly observed him try to inconspicuously slip his seatbelt on.

'Good afternoon, Sir,' said Rowdy, giving his customary greeting, followed by the routine spiel. 'You were observed not wearing your seatbelt. Could I see your driver's licence please?'

The driver was immediately on the offensive. 'I have it on, look!' he said adamantly, as he pulled the seatbelt away from his chest, then let it snap back again.

'I can see that,' said Rowdy with a conscious effort to stay calm. 'But further down the road you were observed not wearing it, and then I observed you putting it on.'

'But I've had it on the whole time,' blurted the driver.

Rowdy was not going to enter into an argument with the man. He knew what he had seen and was confident that Baz was in the same boat.

'Please produce your licence, sir,' said Rowdy. An air of authority attached to his words.

The driver produced his licence, venting his anger towards Rowdy. His frustration turned into uncontrolled abuse as Rowdy calmly issued him with a ticket.

The driver had venom dripping from his words when he said, 'I'll be seeing you in Court over this. It's only your word against mine.'

'That's okay, sir,' replied Rowdy steadily, not allowing himself to be drawn into the abuse. 'I get paid to go to court.'

The driver removed a pen from his top pocket and demanded Rowdy's name. Rowdy graciously obliged by pointing to his name tag and repeated it for the man. Without another word, the driver swung out into the flow of traffic, narrowly missing another vehicle.

Bryan was resting against the bonnet of the police car, grinning smugly as Rowdy approached. 'You realise I haven't had one abusive customer all day.'

'That's easily fixed. Give me your name tag,' Rowdy said, suggesting they swap names.

'Do you remember the days when we didn't have to give out our names, and just had an identification number?' Bryan asked.

'What, the good old days,' recalled Rowdy.

'That's them,' Bryan agreed.

'I do actually. I remember working in the Wild Cattle Creek State Forest, up near Dorrigo, amongst the logging protesters once,' Rowdy recounted with some amusement. 'We used to swap our badge numbers to confuse the protesters.'

Rowdy explained how they would swap their identification number with another officer, who was the opposite in physical appearance. For the most part, they would mingle with the protesters and engage them in civil and social conversation. The media would arrive to report on the situation. Once the cameras were rolling, the placid crowd turned into a raucous, and obnoxious, cauldron of humanity. Their conversations with police was replaced with insulting taunts and spitting. They enjoyed provoking an officer into assaulting them, or using a rough hand in their arrest, knowing full well that the scene would be replayed to the nation on the early news.

Complaints would inevitably be made against police. The subsequent investigation would often stall, however, when it was realised that the protester had incorrectly recorded the officer's identification number, when the description they gave of the officer failed to match the number.

'I'm shocked,' Bryan said in mock disbelief. 'I would never have done anything like that.'

'Hey, I just remembered,' Rowdy said, changing the subject as a name from the past popped into his head. 'Do you remember Sam Drake?'

'Sure do. He worked here for a couple of years,' Bryan answered as he recalled his old work colleague.

'He's getting out of the job,' said Rowdy.

'Hurt on duty?'

'Yeah, he got stabbed during a pub brawl a few months back and has lost the use of an arm,' Rowdy said as easily as if discussing the weather.

'The lucky, lucky bastard,' said Bryan with some jealousy. He had often dreamt of receiving his own HOD pension someday. 'The extent people go to, just to get out of this job.'

The portable radio then crackled and the two officers immediately turned their attention to the approaching traffic to wave down the next vehicle to be called in.

'Anyone else hungry?' crackled the voice of Baz.

1.30PM

Dick had just finished using a paper towel to dry the hands. He walked over to a nearby cabinet with a bold police sticker across its two steel doors. He took hold of both circular handles, turned them simultaneously, and pulled the doors open. Dick removed a bottle of methylated spirits which he use to clean and dry the skin on the hands further.

There are numerous methods used to fingerprint a corpse. Most bodies can be fingerprinted in the same manner as a healthy, living person. Dick was faced with a challenge, though; he was not working with a fresh corpse. The hands were partially decomposed and because of their long exposure to water, the skin had absorbed the fluid like a sponge.

The epidermis layer of skin was badly wrinkled and could tear easily. On most of the fingers, that outer layer of the skin had actually partially detached from the inner layer. Dick knew he could remove this outer layer of skin and find the exact same ridge structure on the dermis layer where the ridge structure originates from, deep down in the skin. The outer layer is simply conforming to the pattern that has developed below it.

Fingerprinting that layer is often used on burn victims. Provided the burns haven't penetrated too deeply, the black, charred, and brittle outer skin can be removed to find a new finger beneath.

Dick removed a scalpel from the police cabinet. Hunched over the severed hands, oblivious now to the desecrated corpse sharing the table, he began to delicately slice into the epidermis skin covering the index finger of the left hand. The swollen skin was easily removed.

Even in the frigid climate of the morgue, Dick had to pause while he lifted a shoulder to the side of his face and caught the bead of sweat that trickled from his hair line.

Dick tried to stretch the skin over his own fingertip, like the gloves he was wearing. The skin tore. He returned to the hand and this time removed the skin covering the middle finger. He gently stretched the white and partly translucent skin once more. This time the skin remained intact.

'Look at that,' Dick exclaimed with satisfaction as he held up his finger covered with another man's skin. He admired it as you would try on a ring. Dick tore another wad of paper towel from its dispenser with his free hand. He dabbed the skin to remove some moisture that had been squeezed out.

Dick chose to lightly apply a fine black powder with a squirrel hair brush to the foreign skin. Whilst precariously holding the skin flap in place over his own left index finger with thumb and middle finger, with his other hand he placed a small, glossy white card against the powdered skin. The black powder was transferred onto the card. To preserve the fingerprint for identification, he covered it with clear tape that was normally used for lifting fingerprints off hard surfaces.

Now that the fingerprint was safely encased between card and tape, Dick retrieved a small magnifying glass from the cabinet and inspected the result. He was happy with what he saw. There were more than sufficient minutiae points to perform a comparison. The detail was so good; Dick could even see tiny white dots along the black powder ridges that were the skins sweat pores.

Dick returned to the hands and started the same process all over again. Of the ten fingers, he only failed to achieve a suitable impression on three. Dick was not aware whether the owner of the hands had a prior fingerprint record, or if forensic police would have to try to develop fingerprints from his belongings. Either way, the more usable prints that Dick could obtain the better.

'How did you do?' a morgue assistant asked as Dick started to pack his equipment.

'Seven out of ten,' Dick boasted, having to raise his voice over the wine of a vibrating saw that the assistant was using to cut the skull cap off the corpse.

'With that strike rate, you'll be back here more often,' the assistant said without pausing from his work.

Dick cringed at the thought. As far as he was concerned, the least amount of time spent at the morgue the better.

He dropped the hands back into the bucket, thanked the morgue assistant and said his goodbyes. He returned to the front room where he had obtained his protective clothing and tossed them into the canvas bins provided.

As Dick stood at the wash basin, scrubbing and disinfecting his hands, his stomach grumbled loudly to make him aware how hungry it was. He contemplated where he would go for lunch. An image flashed into his mind. He pictured himself eating a bread roll. He held the roll with two hands and took a bite. The pleasure he felt as he savoured the taste turned to disgust as he realised that the hands holding the roll were not his own. They were the grotesque severed hands of a corpse. Lunch could wait.

Ricky entered the front station area just as the Station Officer was rising from behind the telephone switchboard to serve a young man standing at the enquiry counter. The small brass bell attached to the top of the wooden entrance door, still tinkled as the door jerked closed.

'Shooters licence,' was all the young man said as he placed both his hands onto the counter top.

Ricky watched as the Station Officer paused and stood, halfway across the room on his journey towards the front counter.

'Here we go,' said Ricky quietly to himself, well aware the Station Officer hated bad manners. Without an introduction, greeting, or cursory hello, the young man will have ticked the bad manners box inside his head.

The Station Officer stood still, just looking at the young man standing at the counter, then resumed his approach to the counter and stood directly opposite the man. He placed his hands on the counter in a mirror image of the young man before him.

With a dead pan face the Station Officer said, 'Elephant.'

A baffled look crossed the young man's face. He remained silent, not knowing how to respond.

The Station Officer replied with enthusiasm, 'It's a word game right? You come in and say a word, and then I have to say the first word that pops into my head.'

The baffled look on the young man's face became one of total confusion. 'Nnn... No, I... I... want to apply for a... shooters licence.'

'Oh, I see... you would like to apply for a Shooters licence,' he continued, placing emphasis on the word *apply*.

The young man again faltered. 'Th ... Th... that's right.'

'Well, not as much fun as a word game, but I can certainly help you to *apply* for a shooters licence.'

The Station Officer removed an application form from a shelf under the counter and explained its completion to the young man, who now spoke in clear sentences. A firearms safety test was produced and the young man paid the required fee. With concentration, he started to circle the appropriate multiple choice answers.

'Any jobs come in while I was tied up with IA?' Ricky asked while the Station Officer continued with the applicant, requesting a criminal history check on the man on his computer.

'Only a stealing,' he replied and searched through the mess of paperwork on his desk. 'Here are the details,' he finally handed Ricky a piece of paper.

'Thanks,' Ricky said to show off his good manners. 'I see you have been entertaining yourself again,' he indicated with a nod, to the young man deep in concentration at the counter.

'You know how it is. Quiet day behind the desk, gets a bit boring,' he explained.

'Are you going to ask this poor bloke the dog question when he completes the test?' Ricky asked, even though he knew what the answer would be.

'Never let a chance go by, a wise man once said.'

'Excuse me,' the young man politely interrupted. 'I've finished the form.'

The Station Officer sprang from his chair and removed the overlay sheet to the multiple choice questions from under the counter. 'Let's see how you've done then,' he said, unable to wipe the grin from his face. 'One-hundred percent correct,' the Station Officer announced as he saw all the man's answers correspond with the template. The young man grinned from ear to ear with his success. 'Don't get too cocky though,' the Station Officer said seriously. 'There's one last question to be answered and if you don't get it correct, your paperwork is stamped never to be issued with a shooters licence.'

The unexpected pressure immediately showed on the young man's face.

Several months ago, the Station Officer had attended a shooting incident on one of the large properties surrounding Chifley. A farmer had been driving an old paddock basher around the property with his blue cattle dog sitting on the bench seat beside him for company. A rifle was propped against the seat between them. The butt of the rifle was on the floor and the barrel pointed skyward, towards the battered roof lining. The dog, in its bid to get comfortable, bumped the rifle, knocking it against the farmer's left arm. The dog then pawed at the rifle, pulling the trigger with a claw. The loaded firearm discharged and shot the farmer in the arm. When the Station Officer arrived, along with the ambulance, all the farmer could do was laugh as he explained, 'Me bloody dog shot me.'

The Station Officer now explained the question to the young man. 'It's a very simple true or false question. If you don't know the answer, you've got a fifty-fifty chance of getting it right anyway.'

'Okay, I'm ready,' said the young man, totally unaware of the set up.

'You should never let a blue cattle dog use a loaded firearm?' said the Station Officer, appearing to read from a formal looking document.

The young man's happy demeanour returned instantly as he realised he was the source of a practical joke.

'You had me worried there for a minute,' he laughed.

The station officer stretched a hand out across the counter which was happily shaken. 'Well done,' congratulated the Station Officer. 'You've passed.' The young man left the station with the knowledge that his shooters licence would be forwarded to him in the mail.

'Had your fun now?' Ricky asked, pushing himself off the wall he had leant on to view the proceedings.

'Yes thanks,' said the Station Officer. 'Now get out of my station and go and do some work. You're making the place look untidy.'

2PM

Rowdy was back in his Highway Patrol car after taking a short meal break. He was patrolling south on the Great North Highway, doing laps of the twenty-five kilometre stretch of road between Benstown and the township of Bowen. Bryan and Baz had paired up, and were patrolling the forty-five kilometres to Brookstone.

An electrical lead was draped over Rowdy's left leg. It had a small plastic hand piece at one end, which was the lock and release control for the microwave speed indicator instrument fitted to the vehicle. The control piece nestled in his lap, ready for use.

The other end of the lead snaked its way towards the front dash, where the computer and display section of the radar was securely fitted in the centre. Mounted outside the vehicle and just behind Rowdy's head, was the radar's antenna. The device was a simple Doppler radar, but extremely accurate. Prior to starting his patrol, Rowdy had performed a series of tests on the device, using musical tuning forks, and found it to be working correctly.

Rowdy approached a crest on the highway. He had patrolled this section of roadway so many times before; he was intimate with every turn, hill, and pothole along its length. Rowdy could already picture the unseen road beyond the crest. Every line marking, signpost, culvert, and tree appeared in his mind as he neared the crest.

It was a section of road that he and his colleagues affectionately referred to as, *the speed bowl*. It was basically, one enormous dish drain, which stretched for three kilometres from crest to crest. It was a popular fishing spot for the local highway constabulary.

Rowdy cleared the northern crest and started to descend its gentle slope. He travelled deeper into the depths of the bowl, only to be disappointed that there was not another vehicle in sight. The fish pond was empty.

A lone vehicle appeared over the distant southern crest. Even at a distance of twenty-five hundred metres, Rowdy estimated the vehicle's speed to be in excess of the one-hundred kilometres an hour limit. He reached down from the steering wheel without even a glance to feel the familiar shape of the remote handpiece nestled in his lap.

Rowdy pushed a button and released the radar's invisible beam. An instant later, two blank windows on the dash mounted computer came to life in brilliant red. The number 98 appeared in the police vehicle's patrol display. Rowdy took a quick glance at the calibrated speedometer of the police vehicle. He saw the indicator gauge only a needle width away from the one-hundred.

Rowdy returned his attention to the approaching bright yellow vehicle, satisfied that the speed recorded by the radar, correlated with that shown on the speedometer of the police car. The target window on the computer section showed the number 119 and was increasing rapidly.

There were no other cars on the road between Rowdy and the target vehicle. Fortunately for Rowdy, no other vehicles had appeared over the southern crest behind the victim he had securely locked in his sights. So far, it was a copy book speed check.

The cabin of Rowdy's vehicle was filled with a screeching noise. To anyone other than a highwayman, it would have been a maddening sound to torture the eardrum. It was music to Rowdy's ears. The sound wave danced on his eardrum as pleasantly as if an orchestra was playing the Blue Danube Waltz. The source of the symphony was the dash mounted radar computer.

The tone it emitted was clear and constant, but increased in pitch, as the number in the target window continued to increase past 125.

'Let's see how long it takes this loser to spot me,' Rowdy said softly to himself, his eyes constantly darting from the approaching car to the computer display.

There was still no other vehicle in sight to interfere with the speed check. There was not even a hint of crackle in the tone to indicate interference of any kind as Rowdy conducted the orchestra with finesse.

Only a three second radar check is sufficient to prove a speeding offence. Rowdy's check had been going for five seconds, and the two vehicles were still two-thousand metres apart and closing. The target display now reached 135 and still increasing, to match the crescendo that was being played by the radar's computer. The tone climaxed when the number display showed 141 and remained steady.

Rowdy was now into his fifteenth second of the speed-check. The two vehicles were within fifteen-hundred metres of one another, with the bright yellow target vehicle maintaining a speed of one-hundred and forty kilometres an hour. The target display was only varying by a kilometre or two, as the offending driver maintained his excessive speed through the speed bowl.

Rowdy was amazed that no other vehicle had appeared in his forward vision. 'He still hasn't spotted me as a fully marked police car,' he again said softly to himself. 'Let's see how long it takes him to remove his head from his arse.'

Now thirty seconds into the speed check, the two vehicles were five-hundred metres apart. The pristine sunny day offered unobstructed vision on the open highway for miles. Rowdy could not believe the driver had failed to see him. He was in a vehicle decorated with red and blue beacons that would glint in the sunlight even when they were not turned on. His Highway Patrol car had numerous large aerials mounted on the roof to catch an observant eye, not to mention the large reflective police sticker across the bonnet.

'His head must be that far up, it's stuck,' Rowdy now thought.

Then it happened. The nose of the approaching vehicle dipped sharply towards the roadway as its driver stood onto the brake pedal. In his haste to slow his speeding vehicle, the driver nearly pushed the brake pedal all the way to the floor. Wheels briefly locked up before the car's computer engaged the anti-lock braking system. The hurtling car slewed from side to side slightly as its chassis absorbed the rapid deceleration. Puffs of light blue smoke from the tyres, spun in the vortex created behind the car.

Rowdy watched the car noticeably slow down, he heard the tone sung by the radar, drop in pitch. The target display plummeted from 140 to 115, at which point Rowdy locked the display with another push of the button on the handpiece.

When one-hundred metres separated the two vehicles, Rowdy activated his blue and red emergency beacons and gave a couple of rapid flicks of the headlights. This was usually enough for most people to realise they had to pull over.

Rowdy had all but stopped his police car when the offending driver passed, by now doing the speed limit. The driver was making no attempt to stop. Rowdy quickly swung his vehicle into a U-turn, just missing the rear bumper of the offender's car. Rowdy now used the full acceleration of his high performance vehicle to take up a position behind the other car. The police siren was yelping and wailing to get the driver's full attention. Still, the offender did not indicate or make a move to pull over.

'We've got a player,' Rowdy said to himself, grabbed the police radio handpiece, and informed the operator of his location and registration number of the offending vehicle. He also requested a stolen check. Rowdy's suspicions were always heightened when it was obvious that an offender was ignoring him. He may be buying more time while he tried to secrete something in the vehicle. He watched intently, to make sure nothing was tossed out the window, or to see if there was any other movement inside the vehicle.

The police radio operator replied seconds after he made the request, relaying the registered owner's details and stating that the vehicle was not reported stolen.

Rowdy knew the vehicle could still be stolen; the owner just did not know it yet.

After travelling a further five-hundred metres, the offending vehicle started to slow and indicated, as it pulled over to the left and stopped. Rowdy cautiously approached the driver who wound his window fully down. Before Rowdy could say anything, the male driver asked, 'How are you, buddy?'

'I'm fine thanks,' replied Rowdy. As soon as Rowdy laid eyes on the driver, he had a familiar feeling that he knew him, but no name popped into his head.

'Sir, your speed was checked on radar at one-hundred and forty kilometres an hour. Can I see your driver's licence please?'

'Certainly,' the driver agreed, calmly and confidently.

Rowdy took the licence and read the man's name. It matched the name he had been given by the radio operator as the registered owner. The name, however, still failed to ring any bells in Rowdy's memory.

'Is there any reason for your speed?' Rowdy asked.

The driver continued his charade. 'I'm sorry, but I didn't realise I was going that fast. My speedo only said one-hundred. It mustn't be working correctly.'

He had heard this excuse countless times before, but more importantly, he now placed that excuse to a face. He knew the driver looked familiar. Rowdy started to dig a little deeper.

'Have you ever been fined before, sir?' asked Rowdy, not letting on that he now recognised the man.

'No. I always drive within the speed limit,' the driver replied.

It all came back to Rowdy. Even the car was matching the face and excuse in Rowdy's memory bank. Six months previously, Rowdy had stopped this same man in Benstown, for a minor speeding offence of seventy-two in a sixty zone. The same confident manner and excuse had been forthcoming then, and Rowdy had let the man off with a caution.

'Have you ever been stopped for speeding before?' Rowdy asked, digging a deeper hole for the man to jump into.

The driver did not hesitate to lie. 'Never, no.'

Rowdy considered explaining the facts of life about his lying and speeding ways, but decided to save his breath. 'You'll be receiving a fine for speeding today. I won't keep you long.'

The driver quickly got out of his car to follow Rowdy back towards the police vehicle. 'That's a bit unfair!' the driver exclaimed to Rowdy's back, with a hint of desperation seeping into his voice. 'I told you, it's not my fault. My speedo must be out.'

Rowdy turned and shot the man a deathly stare before saying with forced restraint, 'That's what you said last time.'

The driver's face became a study of concentration as Rowdy could almost hear the man's mind turning over.

The controlled pleasantness had now gone out of Rowdy's voice when he said, 'I'll help you out. Six months ago, Queen Street, Benstown. Seventy-two in the sixty zone.'

The driver's confident manner crumbled. 'That was you?'

'You're damn right it was me,' Rowdy said aggressively, giving the driver a clear message he was not in the mood to be bounced. 'I'd suggest you sit back in your car and not say another word.'

With all boldness now drained from the driver, he did as he was told and slunk back to his car to await his fate. Shortly Rowdy approached the driver with a handful of tickets. 'The first is for the speed,' explained Rowdy. 'The second is for having that expired registration label on your windscreen and one for the scrubbed out tyre on the back. Steel's showing through the inside shoulder.' He handed over the tickets without explaining any further about their method of disposal. He turned and walked back to his police vehicle, satisfied the motorist had finally got what he deserved. Rowdy had no way of knowing, but this driver was one that sped every day, and would probably continue to.

'Hello, Mr. Harris is it?' Ricky asked of the old man who opened the creaking front door of a time worn weatherboard cottage in the heart of Chifley.

'That's right,' he croaked in a voice that sounded as frail as the front door looked.

The eighty-year old man struggled to straighten from his arthritic hunch as he pushed on a walking stick held in his shaking right hand. His face rose to see the two police officers standing on his veranda. The toughened and wrinkled skin on his face showed the marks of a lifetime spent under the sun. The weathered features, however, could not disguise the vibrant blue eyes, which still shone as brightly as a lighthouse lamp. They revealed a man who lived a happy, fulfilled, and contented life.

Ricky held the flimsy fly screen door open and was surprised the old man offered his hand to shake after transferring his walking stick to the other. When the old man first opened the door, Ricky had made the conscious decision not to extend his own hand in greeting – not out of rudeness, but in consideration of the man's infirm appearance.

'You rang and reported a tree stolen,' said Ricky as their hands met. Ricky was astonished at the firmness in the old man's grip. The hard calloused hand, with its thick fingers, consumed his; the man's forearm still dense with muscle from a lifetime of labour.

'That's right,' quivered the old man's voice. 'Someone stole my Chinese Tallow-wood.'

'If it's not too much trouble, can you show me where it was taken from, please?'

'No trouble at all lad.' The old man raised his walking stick and used it as a pointer. 'Just out the front here,' he said as he shuffled across the threshold.

Ricky and Tombstone had to quickly stand to either side to let him pass. They were both amazed at the stooped man's turn of speed. The two officers followed as the old man barely slowed to descend the handful of steps from the veranda into the front yard.

The aging house was surrounded by manicured lawn. Garden beds were full of flowering colour, interspersed with textured foliage plants and shapely shrubs.

Ricky admired the garden's charm and elegance. 'You certainly have a beautiful garden Mr. Harris.'

The old man walked off the meandering pathway and onto the lawn. 'Oh, it's not my garden lad. It's my wife's,' he said proudly and raised the walking stick again to wave it in a sweeping motion around the garden.

'She must spend hours in it,' commented Ricky, as he struggled to find just one weed game enough to stick its head up.

A shadow briefly passed over the old man's eyes, dulling their brilliance. 'My wife passed away twenty-five years ago.'

Ricky immediately felt embarrassed for his unintentional insensitive comment. 'I'm sorry,' he said sheepishly.

The old man's eyes cleared and their rich glow returned as he took comfort in the memory of his forty-five years of marriage.

'I've been taking care of her life's passion ever since,' he said and smiled.

Even though the old man had lost his wife all that time ago, Ricky still felt that uneasiness of what to say. 'She would no doubt be proud of your efforts,' he managed to utter.

The old man walked to the centre of the lawn on one side of the path and taped his walking stick onto the manicured grass several times. 'The tree was here.'

With a bewildered look, Ricky looked down at the lush, green grass. There was no vacant hole or dishevelled mound of dirt with broken off roots to indicate a plant of any kind had been removed.

'I planted that tree sixty years ago,' the old man explained. His eyes began to swell with tears. 'The day after we got back from our honeymoon, my wife and I planted it when this place was nothing but weeds.'

'But there's…' Ricky started to say, but was quickly cut short when Tombstone stepped from behind him and placed a heavy hand on his shoulder. Tombstone moved forward as he pulled on Ricky's shoulder.

Tombstone had not said a word the entire time. He was letting his young offsider take charge of this simple stealing report. Hearing that Ricky was about to inform the old man that there was no evidence of a tree ever being planted there, he was compelled to step in.

'When did you last see the tree, Mr. Harris?' asked Tombstone.

'Last evening,' replied the old man. 'I sit on the veranda every evening to have a cup of coffee and admire its graceful limbs.'

'Looking at that tree must bring back a lot of memories.'

'That tree saw my wife and I raise three children,' the old man said as he looked up through moist blurry eyes, as if following the trunk of the tree to its branches.

Ricky watched in silence, still trying to fathom out what was going on.

To add to his confusion, Tombstone removed his pen and notebook from a breast pocket and started to record the details of the stealing. Tombstone's finally fallen off the perch, Ricky thought to himself as he watched on bewildered.

'And how tall was the tree Mr. Harris?' asked Tombstone, with his pen poised above the notebook ready to record the answer.

The old man again raised the walking stick and this time pointed towards the roof of the cottage. 'It was a good ten feet above there.'

'It would have shaded the house nicely in the afternoon,' stated Tombstone as he now pictured the majestic old tree.

Ricky nearly choked out loud as he watched his deranged partner look up into the vacant sky.

'Nature's own air conditioning my wife used to call it,' laughed the old man at the memory.

Tombstone then spent another ten minutes asking the man questions and obtained a detailed description of the tree. All of which, to Ricky's dismay, Tombstone recorded in his notebook.

Tombstone returned the notebook to his pocket. 'I can't promise you anything Mr. Harris, but we'll do whatever we can to find your tree.'

'I just hope whoever stole it kept enough soil on the roots to keep it alive,' the old man said with genuine concern.

Tombstone gave another look towards the ground and then gave his expert horticultural opinion. 'By the look of that hole, I think they did.'

Ricky nearly fell over as he continued to watch the bizarre pantomime. Just to be sure, though, he could not stop himself from taking another studied look at the ground, just in case he was really missing something.

Ricky and Tombstone were about to leave when the old man insisted they wait, just a minute. He returned inside his home and then reappeared with a bag overflowing with fresh vegetables from his garden in the backyard and handed them to Ricky. He then snapped the stem of a rose bud that was just about to burst into full bloom and held it towards Tombstone.

'I see you're married,' the old man said, using his walking stick to point at the wedding band on Tombstone's finger. 'For your wife,' and gestured the rose towards Tombstone again.

Tombstone took the rose from the old man's shaking hand. 'Thank you very much.' The big burly policeman then raised the rose bud to his nose and inhaled its sweet perfume.

A spark then flashed from the old man's eyes when he said with a wink, 'You may even get lucky tonight.'

The two police officers sat back in their vehicle. Tombstone's face still flushed from the old man's parting remark.

'Would you mind telling me what just happened,' said Ricky.

Tombstone delicately placed the rose into the bag of vegetables. 'It's obvious, isn't it?' he said with surprise that Ricky had not caught on. 'The old bloke is obviously suffering from dementia.'

'For a minute there I thought you were too,' replied Ricky.

'In his mind, a tree was stolen,' explained Tombstone. 'When I put the incident report in, I'll cross the doubtful box.'

What Ricky and Tombstone could not know was the old man did plant a tree when he and his wife were married, sixty years ago. The day after she died, a severe storm hit the town and uprooted the tree which then had to be removed. In his aging years, the old man's faculties were now failing him. He would sit on his veranda and his mind's eye would see that grand tree in his front yard as a connection to his wife. In a partially lucid moment, he must have seen the tree was gone and assumed someone stole it.

Hopefully tomorrow, he will see that the tree has been located by police and replanted, so he can again sit every evening and admire it, and enjoy the memories that are connected with it.

After retrieving his gun and returning the locker key to the morgue receptionist, Dick made the short, one block walk to Kingstown Hospital where his father had been admitted.

At seventy-nine years of age, his father had suffered numerous health issues over the years. Having been a heavy smoker from a young age, it was not surprising that twenty-five years ago his family GP gave the news to either stop smoking or have his leg amputated. The shock of that day was enough to ensure he never placed another cigarette to his mouth. He also managed to keep his leg by replacing his blocked artery with that of a pig.

The years since had not been illness free. There was heart surgery to again clear arteries blocked by the effects of smoking and cholesterol issues. The constant battle against diabetes ensured his diet was at least improved. It was only the last few years that medication was required to keep it in check. He survived prostate cancer and was one of the few to survive a melanoma for nearly twenty years now. His latest illness, however, was a mystery. He had countless blood tests and scans, all of which kept coming back negative. Nothing was showing as abnormal to suggest a reason for his current ill health. Dick often wondered whether he had just chosen that this was the time for his life to end. Not that he had given up on life, but had got to the stage where he had accomplished his life's goals. He had lived with the loneliness that being a widower brings. He had raised his three children to adulthood and was now the proud grandfather of nine. Perhaps he considered it was now time to pass the baton on to Dick and his two brothers, for they had now become their father's generation.

Dick was constantly reminded in his thoughts and nightmares that death can come prematurely for many. It can come suddenly, violently, and without choice. If this *choice* was in fact the case with his father, then it spoke volumes of the man he was. To face that natural fear of death, head on, takes courage and faith.

Dick walked down the hospital corridor, forcing himself to smile pleasantly to patients and other visitors who stared at his uniform.

Even though he knew the room, Dick still counted down the room numbers displayed above each door. He walked into the private room to find him propped up in bed, fast asleep.

Someone was sitting beside the bed, his face hidden by an opened newspaper. On hearing Dick's footsteps, the newspaper was lowered to reveal his eldest brother, Stewart.

'I didn't expect it to be you, Dick,' Stewart said with surprise.

'Hi Stu,' said Dick, crossing the room to shake his brothers hand. 'How is he?'

'I've only been here half an hour, but he seemed pretty good. He's only just fallen off to sleep.'

Dick leaned on the rail at the foot of the bed as his brother relaxed again into his chair. 'Any more tests today?' asked Dick.

Stewart reached out and rolled the small table that was across his father's bed to one side. 'Not today. I checked with the nurses and there hasn't been any other test results come back either.'

Dick lifted up the medical chart hanging on the end of the bed and flicked through the pages. The only sense he could make of them was the line graph that recorded his father's blood pressure.

'What brings you down this way besides dad?' Dick's brother asked.

Dick returned the medical chart. 'I had a quick job at the morgue. It was a bit of a handful but all went well,' said Dick, without sharing further details. He then grabbed another chair and moved it to the same side of the bed his brother was sitting. 'What about you?' asked Dick, changing the subject. 'Work going okay?'

'Everything's fine. I only spend two days a week in Sydney at the moment, so that's a bonus.'

Their father stirred and moaned briefly before settling back to sleep. The top of the bed was raised up with their father nestled in a cluster of pillows. His stirring had caused his head to tilt to one side and his mouth opened slightly. His bottom dentures were dislodged out of place and hung crookedly over his bottom lip, pushed forward by his tongue.

Dick was shocked at the sight and had to avert his eyes. He looked up to study the ceiling, then again glimpsed at his father. His gaze only lasted a second before he again had to look away, repulsed at what he saw. This time he looked at the floor to study the pattern in the tiles.

Dick's hands were in his lap and he noticed they were shaking. Sweat was starting to bead amongst the hairs on the back of them. He again glanced quickly at his father, but the same image was still there.

Dick no longer saw his father. He only saw a twisted and distorted face. He could now feel his heart racing as it tried to pound its way through his chest. Sweat oozed from every pore in his body. Stewart noticed his brother's agitation. 'Are you alright?'

Dick's voice trembled, 'All I see is a gunshot to the head.' He looked everywhere but at his father.

It took a moment before Stewart realised what was happening. 'It's okay. Dad is just asleep.'

'But the mouth, the distortion in his face,' Dick tried to explain. His anxiety worsened and he started to wring his hands together. His body rocked back and forth as sweat now trickled down his face and back. No matter where he looked, or if he closed his eyes, the bloodied, distorted, and disfigured head of a gunshot victim was there to taunt him.

'I have to go,' Dick said and abruptly rose from his chair. 'I have to get out of here.'

Dick gave his brother a quick hug. 'Look after him,' were his parting words as he fled the room in a full blown panic attack.

His pace quickened down the corridor the closer he got to the exit. The sliding doors that led outside to the front of the hospital were in sight. Dick all but ran the last few metres. He burst out into the sunshine, oblivious to everything around him. He sat on a low brick retaining wall that doubled as a garden bed. Spreading his legs, he draped his body forward and placed his elbows on his knees to support his upper body. His forearms and hands hung, trembling between his legs, as he tried to will the bad thoughts to go away.

2.30PM

The panic attack that had overwhelmed Dick when visiting his father had subsided, and he now started his drive back towards Brookstone. However his mind still raced through images of the past, flickering like a kaleidoscope of old movie trailers, complete with sound effects and even smells.

Everything around him triggered a memory. He drove past a park full of laughing children enjoying a birthday party. The birthday boy was blindfolded and trying to hit a papier-mâché piñata, formed in the shape of a clown. It was suspended from a swing set frame with a cord tied around its neck like a hangman's noose. It dangled and swayed gently in the breeze as the child was spun around before attempting to strike it. What should have been a happy scene before Dick's eyes was lost in the dark recesses of his mind, where every hanging he had attended over the years replaced it.

He saw bodies hanging in lounge rooms and sheds, while others were in bushland. Just like the birthday party in the park, he had even attended a suicide where the victim had used a swing frame as the suspension point to successfully end their life.

The most horrifying sight, Dick recalled, was a full human pelt hanging in a doorway to dry, after its former wearer had been skinned following their murder. Dick physically shuddered from the thought.

He was now aware he was stopped at traffic lights, as his wandering mind lifted out of its dark haze. He could not remember seeing the lights turning red. Shocked by the lack of alertness to his surroundings, Dick attempted to force the images from his mind, or at least into a dark corner of it. 'Look for the green light,' he said over and over to himself, in an attempt to keep his concentration on driving.

A motorcyclist stopped at the red light in the lane beside him. The traffic lights were instantly gone, as his thoughts scattered across scenes of crumpled and twisted metal that once resembled motorbikes. Every motorbike once had a rider. Those riders who did not lay broken, mangled, and motionless on the roadway, never to breathe again, lay in screaming agony as splintered bones tore through skin and clothing.

The roar of the motorbike as it accelerated away startled Dick. He now saw the green light and sedately pulled away, willing himself to stay alert. He turned up the volume on the commercial radio, just like he had done earlier in the day to help keep his mind in the present. It failed to work. Dick was lost again as the radio announcer was reminding his listeners Christmas was not far away. All he heard now was the uncontrolled sobbing of a mother who had just run over her two-year old daughter.

It was Christmas morning. Mum was a nurse and had just finished opening presents with her young family before leaving for work. As she reversed down her driveway, she failed to see her excited two year old run from the house. Believing all her children were safe inside the house, she was surprised at the dull thud at the back of her car. Before she could stop, she heard a crunching sound as a rear wheel rolled over something.

Dick's vision turned red as he watched the blood congeal on the concrete driveway around the crushed head of a two year old little girl. Christmas Day was not meant to be like this; he saw himself storming into the nearest church, interrupting the morning Christmas Service, and conveying the minister to the young couples home to give whatever comfort their faith could bring.

148

The red that blanketed his vision then began to fade as rivulets of blood were hosed down the driveway into the gutter.

Anger rose inside Dick. The rage that swelled was directed towards himself. He questioned what right he had to feel affected by these events. His family was still safe, as was he. How did those directly involved in these horrific trials resume any normality to life? They are the ones that need the help, not me, Dick would tell himself as he again denied he had a problem.

Tombstone returned the radio handpiece to its cradle on the dash of Chifley 10. 'What better way to end the day,' he said as he turned his head and smiled at Ricky in the driver's seat. Tombstone had just acknowledged the radio message to attend a hanging in bushland, on the town's outskirts. He assumed suicide, and quietly prayed it was nothing more sinister. There was nothing worse than a simple death, made more complicated by murder.

Ricky continued to head towards the police station. 'We knock off in one hour. Can't we leave it for the arvo shift?'

Tombstone quickly considered the request, and then as equally and swiftly, dismissed it. 'No, it happened on our shift. It's our job,' he replied, with a finality in his voice that Ricky failed to pick up on.

'I'm sure he won't mind hanging around another hour.'

Tombstone replied with a firm, 'No', and ignored Ricky's attempts at humour.

Ricky persisted. 'But I'm playing squash at four.'

Tombstone hated being left jobs from a previous shift, so he was not going to do the same to someone else. 'No,' he again replied, this time in such a tone that left Ricky in no doubt the conversation was over. He indicated his defeat by putting on the right blinker of the police truck and turned away from the police station. They drove the next ten minutes in complete silence until one of those rare events occurred, Tombstone actually instigated a conversation.

'Did you know I did a hanging in gaol once?' he said. He settled back into his seat and rested his head back.

'I thought that would be a fairly common place for hangings,' replied Ricky.

'It is,' acknowledged Tombstone. 'But this one happened only fifty centimetres above the ground.'

'How did he manage that?' he asked.

'It was here in Chifley Gaol,' Tombstone vividly recalled. 'He secured a torn bed sheet to the rail of his bed head with the other end around his neck, obviously. Its length was short enough so when he lay on the ground, his neck and head were suspended. Enough weight was exerted on the ligature to slowly choke him.'

'He was determined,' said Ricky, as he tried to visualise how a person could do such a thing. 'I think I would get to the point where it hurt and I would have to sit up.'

'Makes you consider what type of dark place a person would have to be in to go through with it,' pondered Tombstone.

Ricky briefly considered his own happiness and well being. He could not recall ever being in such a dark place where he would even contemplate such an act. Sure, he got down sometimes, but would quickly pick himself up, dust himself off, and get back to enjoying life.

The whole concept of suicide or self-harm was totally foreign to him. It was right up there next to his views and knowledge of depression and other psychological illnesses. 'I'm damned sure I'd never do it.'

Tombstone considered telling Ricky a few facts about life, but instead remained silent. He decided to let his young offsider learn from experience, rather than be forced to listen to the ramblings of an old senior constable, who had experienced more than any person should have to. 'I'll check back with you in twenty years' time on that one,' Tombstone said, somewhat ambiguously.

Ricky accelerated past several slower vehicles. Tombstone raised his left hand and grabbed onto the small handle located just above the door near his head. Tombstone always found it a little unnerving sitting in the passenger seat with someone else in charge of the controls, and his fate. Tombstone again started a conversation to take his mind off Ricky's driving. 'I've only ever done male hangings,' he said. Ricky glanced across at his partner while overtaking another vehicle. 'You watch the road,' Tombstone added, pointing towards the windscreen. 'I'll do the looking around.'

Ricky looked back towards the front.' Well, stop surprising me by all this jovial conversation. I'm starting to think you like me.'

'Well, think about it?' continued Tombstone. 'Have you ever seen, or heard, of a female hanging themselves?'

'Can't say that I have,' replied Ricky.

Silence filled the cabin again as Tombstone pondered the thought briefly, and then added, 'Someone has probably done a study on that very anomaly.'

Ricky turned off the bitumen onto a dirt track that led into sparse bushland just south of town. 'Sounds like someone who needs to find a hobby,' he said as the police truck bounced through culverts and shuddered over the corrugated surface.

'Do you need to take another break?' Lynda asked her husband as they approached the outskirts of Bowen.

'I'm feeling fine,' Lindsay replied as he checked the time on the dashboard clock to see how long he had been driving. 'We'll keep pushing on.'

The roadway had narrowed again to single lanes as they drove over White Creek, just on the northern approach to Bowen. The dual-lane divided concrete carriageway, which had stretched for the last ten kilometres, began to shrink away in Lindsay's rear vision mirror as the couple pushed on towards Sydney.

The new section of road that was left behind had replaced a notorious black spot known as the Telford Bends. It was once a narrow road that twisted and curved its way through a dense section of bushland and was the scene of countless fatal collisions. It used to be a section of road that had few distinguishable landmarks, except for one. Accidents would always be described as north or south of the *bikini tree*. The bikini tree was a big old eucalypt whose growth over the years managed to produce some irregularities in its trunk. One of the locals, or regular commuters along the section of old highway, had obviously studied the tree in worrying detail. They had noticed that it resembled the female form. Pink paint was then applied to accentuate the appropriate bulges and contours to reveal a rather attractive, well-endowed tree wearing bikini top and bottom.

Lindsay pushed a button on his door. An electric motor whirled as the glass window disappeared into the door frame.

'I can drive some of the way if you're feeling tired,' Lynda said as she rubbed a caring hand on her husband's arm.

'Really, I'm feeling fine. It beats sitting on the tractor all...' Lindsay's voice was instantly lost in the shattering of glass.

The couples lives, future, hopes, and dreams were instantly shattered along with their cars windscreen.

Rowdy had fished out the speed bowl he had been patrolling. Checking the time, he started to patrol further south towards Bowen. He was due to knock off in an hour. He would pick his kids up from school in Bowen at three, and then return to Benstown to get them to their dental appointment.

With his shift all but over, a sense of calm encased him at the thought of another working day coming to an end. The insulation from the outside world that the capsule of his highway car offered, added to his security. Nothing could interfere with his day now.

Rowdy crossed White Creek where it trickled under the Great North Highway. His upbeat mood soon soured, as up ahead, he spotted a woman standing very close to the roadway. She was near the back of a car stopped in the breakdown lane with her hands raised, waving above her head.

As Rowdy approached closer, the woman began to jump up and down excitedly while still waving her hands back and forth across each other.

'What does this idiot want?' Rowdy growled, as the bubble he had just created around himself popped.

Mel Folson was just on her way into Bowen. She was travelling alone and had been following the same car for the last fifteen kilometres. She was just commenting to herself how refreshing it was to see another motorist obeying all the road rules, and then suddenly, the vehicle in front swerved violently, just as a semi-trailer travelling in the opposite direction passed them both.

Mel noticed there were two people in the vehicle, but didn't see anything happen inside the vehicle, or outside for that matter, to suggest a reason for the unexpected manoeuvre. She immediately assumed a tyre must have blown, which caused the vehicle to swerve towards the centre line, then back across the edge line. She started to brake, creating some distance between her own car and the erratic, weaving car ahead.

Looking through the rear windscreen of the car in front, Mel noticed the passenger was leaning across towards the driver and appeared to be wrestling with the steering wheel. Mel thought the couple must be having some sort of domestic dispute and she became more determined to distance herself from the other vehicle.

Mel watched on as the vehicle in front started to slow and jerk its way further to the left, into the breakdown lane. Mel continued to reduce her own speed to match but stayed within her lane. The erratic vehicle now came to a complete stop.

Mel had an appointment to get to and was just about to start accelerating again to pass the vehicle when her caring nature got the better of her. Putting on her left blinker, she pulled over and stopped two car lengths behind. Cautious, and not wanting to place herself in danger, Mel remained in her car and focused intently on the what was going on inside the other vehicle. The passenger, who she could now see was female, was still leaning across towards the driver.

When Mel opened her door, she immediately heard the high pitched screams of a distraught woman. Without any further consideration to her safety, Mel raced to the front passenger door of the vehicle in front.

The window was up, but the screams of the frantic woman inside were still ear piercing.

Mel tapped a finger on the outside of the glass. 'Is everything alright,' she asked, but it was clear that it was not.

The woman inside the car was blinded, by sheer terror, to Mel's presence. From her standing position outside the car, Mel's vision of the driver was obscured by the roof. She now bent down to again wrap her knuckles on the side window, but was brought up short.

She now saw the full horror inside the vehicle. Her innocent eyes that would never view the world in the same light again widened. She froze, immediately feeling nauseated, and her legs threatened to give way. She stumbled towards the rear of the car as she attempted to straighten, falling against the car for support.

Trying to calm the hysteria that was welling within her, Mel asked herself what to do, only to have it rush out as her own scream.

'Oh my God. I have to get help,' she continued to scream, staggering in a daze back towards her own car. 'Mobile phone. Call triple zero.' She told herself what to do, as if following someone else's instructions.

As Mel neared her own car, she noticed another vehicle approaching. She started to wave her hands wildly above her head.

'Help,' she screamed, as if the driver could hear her. 'Help. Please stop.'

The approaching vehicle slowed. Through the fog in Mel's mind she could now see that it was a police vehicle. The prospect of real help now excited her and she began to jump up and down as she waved.

Just prior to the shattering of their windscreen, Lindsay and Lynda had taken no notice of the semi-trailer travelling towards them. Then again, why would they? It was no different from the innumerable others that they had passed on their long journey.

The large prime mover was towing a flatbed trailer. The driver travelled this highway five days a week, delivering his load to the port in Kingstown every day. The twenty-two wheeler was now empty and on its return trip home.

After unloading in Kingstown, the driver had folded and packed his tarps used to cover and secure his load on the journey to the port, in a neat bundle at one end of the trailer.

The driver had done this every day for the last two years that he had been doing this regular run. He had the routine down pat. Today, however, his routine was interrupted. He had finished tensioning up the ratchet strap securing his folded tarps when a foreman at the dockside approached him to double check an item on the load's manifest.

The driver had been using a solid, round, steel bar on the ratchet strap to gain extra leverage and tension. The metal bar was thirty millimetres in diameter, sixty centimetres in length and weighed about three kilograms. When finished tensioning the strap, he would always return the bar into a locked toolbox mounted under the trailer. Today, he placed it onto the hardwood decking of the open sided trailer as he went to speak with the foreman. When he returned to his truck, he gave the metal bar no further thought, climbing straight into the cabin of his rig.

For fifty-five kilometres, the bar had rolled and bounced over the floor of the trailer. Just north of Bowen, the semi-trailer rumbled over a broken and potholed section of roadway, not far from where the road widened into a newly constructed dual lane concrete carriageway.

The heavy sprung suspension on the truck designed to carry forty tonne, barely moved as the large pneumatic tyres bounced their way over the deepening potholes. The metal bar was hurled into the air for the last time, and failed to land back on the trailer.

Lindsay and Lynda didn't even see the lethal object spearing through the air. The metal bar pierced the glass windscreen of their car. The sound of shattering glass was so unexpected that Lynda jumped, from both shock and fright. Lindsay was not so fortunate. He had no time to be shocked, or frightened. He did not react at all as one end of the bar speared into his head like an arrow shot from a bow. The bar struck him in the middle of his forehead, as accurately as if he had a bull's eye painted between his eyebrows and hairline, directly in line with his nose. Skin and bone was no match for the deadly missile as it continued on its trajectory unimpeded. It only stopped when it reached the padded headrest behind Lindsay's head.

Now hysterical, she looked at her husband. The car was driverless at ninety kilometres an hour and swerved out of control. Although she was screaming uncontrollably, she still had the presence of mind to lean out of her seatbelt and reach across to the steering wheel.

Everything was just a blur through the shattered windscreen and she struggled to keep the vehicle travelling in a straight line. She reached down with one hand and found the handbrake lever. She pulled it on slowly and felt the car slow immediately.

Lynda managed to bring the car to a complete stop and made a perfect blind park in the breakdown lane. With shaking hands that were numb with fear, Lynda fumbled to release her seatbelt. The attempt was made more difficult as she strained against the buckle in her haste to get closer to her husband. The instant the clasp released, she sprang up onto the seat, kneeling sideways and grabbed her husband's head that was split in two, with both hands. She incoherently screamed for help.

Rowdy still cursed at the woman waving her arms for him to stop. He passed the two parked cars as he continued to brake, and pulled up about three car lengths in front. He assumed the two cars had been involved in a collision, but a quick glance as he had passed did not reveal any obvious panel damage to the front or rear of either.

Rowdy walked slowly towards the cars and could see now that the first had a shattered front windscreen. The glass was shattered in a circular pattern on the driver's side and spiralled out like a spider's web around a small circular hole. The once clear glass was now a shattered, opaque canvas that blocked his view inside the vehicle.

'Some people get excited about a smashed windscreen,' Rowdy murmured to himself as he approached, and concluded that was what the lady was waving her arms about. Then he heard the screams.

Mel ran down the left side of her car towards Rowdy. 'You have to help him,' she screamed, and pointed towards the other car.

'I have to be a glazier now,' Rowdy's thoughts mumbled at the disturbance to his day, unaware of the tragedy inside the vehicle.

He neared the car and looked through the open driver's window. Rowdy slumped, emotionally and physically, as he was overwhelmed with a familiar feeling of utter helplessness. After a short pause while he analysed what to do, he turned and walked slowly back towards his police vehicle. There was no urge to run. He felt no urgency to contact police radio and notify them of the situation. In his mind, there was no emergency here. The only desire he felt at this point was to get back into his vehicle and drive away. There was nothing he could do to help.

3PM

'Well he certainly looks dead,' Ricky said flatly as he stood and looked up at the body dangling from a tree limb. It was difficult to gauge, but the man would have been in his early thirties. The thick, coarse rope constricted his neck so tightly that skin bulged over it and obscured its full diameter. The man's swollen head tilted acutely to one side. He gazed down at the two officers through bloodshot eyes that threatened to pop from their sockets. The blue lips matched the lividity of his skin. They were parted slightly to reveal a swollen tongue.

The axis bone in his neck had been dislocated, which had severed the spinal cord. Blood pressure to his brain would have instantly dropped, resulting in unconsciousness. The man would no longer feel anything while brain death took several minutes to occur. He would have been completely dead in fifteen minutes, as the rest of his organs shut down.

Tombstone stood beside his young offsider. Both were motionless, with their chins raised and heads cocked to opposite sides.

'Did you know that hanging is still a legal method of judicial execution in sixty countries?' said Tombstone.

'You're just full of useful facts today,' Ricky replied. He raised a hand to shield his eyes from the glare as he continued to look up.

The victim had chosen the middle of a small dirt clearing to carry out his final act. He parked his compact four-wheel-drive under a tree limb that stretched out over the clearing. After leaving a brief hand written note on the driver's seat, he tied one end of a hemp rope to the bull bar of the vehicle. He then climbed onto the vehicle, leaving dents in the thin panels of the bonnet and roof as he went. He then tossed the rope over the sturdy limb and calmly set the ligature in place around his neck and to one side, under his jaw. No doubt without a moment's hesitation, he walked off the side of the roof to his death.

The man fell under a metre until the rope stretched to a neck breaking stop. His body convulsed violently, but was soon reduced to an involuntary twitch. Calmness then followed. The body only swayed, as the gentle breeze tried to caress life back into it.

Ricky became aware the bushland surrounding them was silent. Not a bird, animal, or insect could be heard. It was as if all life around them had ended when the rope snapped taut. The two officers were not only silently watched by the haunting stare of a dead man, but also by every living creature that called this bushland their home. It was as if they could sense a disruption to their ordered world. Ricky shuddered as a tingling sensation passed through him. He closed his eyes, the silence so overwhelming he suddenly had the scary thought he and Tombstone were the only living things left on earth. A relieved smile quickly spread across his face as he heard the rustle of tree tops in the breeze. The rhythmic creaking of rope as it rubbed across bark under the strain of the swaying body added to the growing sounds as the bushland came back to life.

A dull thud caused Ricky to open his eyes. The man's boots struck the side of the small four-wheel-drive as the body now twisted in the strengthening breeze. Ricky could now see the army of ants marching down the length of rope from the branch above. They were quick to take advantage of this fresh source of food that nature offered. The ants swarmed across unblinking eyes and into open cavities. Their mandibles starting to tear into the soft tissue they found. The cycle of life continued.

'Are you all right?' asked Tombstone, cocking an eyebrow towards Ricky.

Ricky, relieved that Tombstone was not his only source of company left in the world, replied, 'Yeah, I just caught a glimpse of a hideous sight for a moment.'

Tombstone, unaware Ricky was talking about him said, 'It could have been worse.'

Ricky was startled. What could be worse than having only Tombstone for company?

Tombstone then continued which clarified his comment. 'He could have got the drop wrong,' and pointed at the distance between the tree-limb and were the man dangled.

Ricky's thoughts were now back on the task at hand. 'What happens if they get it wrong?'

'If the drop is too long,' explained Tombstone, 'then the rope can slice through and decapitate the person. If it's too short, they just thrash around, slowly strangling.'

'Just another of your useful facts?' asked Ricky.

'It's like anything you do in life,' continued Tombstone. 'You may as well try to do it well.'

'I'm sure his family will be comforted to know he did a good job hanging himself.'

'Speaking of family, let's find out who this poor sod is,' said Tombstone seriously. 'I'll search the car. You can search him. Check for any other wounds, too. Let's make sure this is a suicide.'

Lindsay Crisp certainly had more than his cholesterol to worry about now as his body unconsciously battled against death. His heart and lungs struggled on by some primitive reflex, no longer directed to function from brain impulses.

Rowdy had not driven away. He was standing back at the open driver's window after notifying police radio of the situation. He had made the return walk back to Lindsay's car as slowly as possible.

During the journey, he stretched on a pair of latex gloves, whilst quietly wishing to himself that the driver was dead when he got there.

Lindsay's chest heaved as his lungs struggled with every inhale. The moaning sound that accompanied each breathe took Rowdy back to another time and place. The gargling exhale was lower in pitch, as if his lungs were relieved to complete another cycle.

Rowdy did not have to check for a pulse. It was visually apparent his heart was beating strongly as blood oozed from his open head on each constriction of the dying muscle. Lindsay's skull was split in two by the metal bar. Each half splayed open like a wedge to reveal what little brain matter there was left. The open cavity swelled with blood, then seeped down to cover Lindsay's face. All around the inside of the car was splattered with blood. Meaty tissue and brain matter hung from the roof lining like stalactites. Jagged white skull fragments were embedded in the upholstered headrest like Chinese throwing stars.

'Please help him,' Lynda pleaded in between heavy sobs. Her screaming had now stopped. 'You have to help my husband.'

Rowdy's mind just roared, 'What do you want me to do. He's going to die.'

The distress in Lynda's tear soaked face prevented him from uttering these words. Unable to deny her pleading eyes, Rowdy reached in and took hold of each side of Lindsay's head and brought the two halves together and said, 'I'll do what I can.'

A hint of a smile then broke through Lynda's suffering as she whispered, 'Thank you.'

Rowdy stood with his arms stretched inside the vehicle. He looked up and down the highway in both directions, silently pleading for the appearance or sound of an ambulance. He spotted Mel standing near her car.
She had both hands clasped to her face as if trying to block out the horrific view.

With his hands occupied on Lindsay's head, blood oozing through his fingers, Rowdy could not point in Mel's direction. Instead he bored his eyes into her and yelled, 'You,' to get her attention. 'Come and get this woman out of the car.'

Mel hesitantly edged forward and looked around for someone else to take her place, but there was no one else.

'Now,' Rowdy bellowed in frustration to get her moving quicker.

Mel quickened her pace and opened the front passenger door. Lynda climbed out stiffly from a numbness that threatened to paralyse her and was met by Mel's supportive arms. As she straightened, Lynda looked across the roofline of the car and again gave a faint, quivering smile towards Rowdy.

'Is he going to be okay?' she asked.

Rowdy did not know what to say. He knew the man was dying and there was nothing he could do to stop that. Deep down, he knew that the woman asking this question knew its answer as clearly as he did. For the moment, though, she was clutching onto any hope that the inevitable would not happen. In her eyes, Rowdy was that hope.

'He's still alive,' was all Rowdy could feebly come up with.

Rowdy spotted an item of white clothing in the car. 'Toss me that jumper on the floor,' he said to Mel, before she led Lynda away.

Rowdy wrapped the knitted jumper around Lindsay's head in a futile attempt to stem the blood flow. He continued to hold Lindsay's head, applying as much pressure as his hands could exert. Lindsay's head was sagged forward so Rowdy eased it backwards to provide a better airway. He was then flooded with self-doubt as he questioned his action. By giving maximum head tilt, was Lindsay now going to drown in his own blood? Rowdy again looked pleadingly down the highway for help.

Rowdy looked back at Lindsay. The man's breathing was still laboured. 'Shit,' he said as the reality struck him. 'The kids. I'm late to pick them up. Shit. The dentist appointment. Shit. The school play tonight. Shit. Emma's going to kill me.'

Rowdy looked down at the mobile phone that bulged in his pocket. He looked up again at his bloodied hands. The frustration of not being able to use his mobile phone to contact his wife soon left him as he watched Lindsay's chest fall for the last time. The exhale this time was long and effortless. Rowdy willed the chest to rise again. It did not – Lindsay was silent. Rowdy took a red, slimy hand from the blood soaked jumper and felt his neck for a pulse. He searched in vain.

Rowdy looked back at Mel and the woman she cradled in her arms. He could not let go of Lindsay's head and walk away. He wanted her to maintain hope for a little longer. The more selfish reason was that he did not have the strength to tell her that her husband was dead.

His mind now started to race as he questioned how all this happened. Rowdy was unaware of the truck and metal bar. He didn't even know who this person he held was.

How did their lives become entwined? Did this person leave early on his journey or was he running late? He had no answers to the questions that flooded him. In the end, it didn't matter. The result would not change. The question's purpose only served to pass the time of day.

A siren could be heard in the distance. Rowdy turned towards Bowen as an ambulance floated over a crest into view. Help was nearly here.

Dick's galloping thoughts and images from the past now settled somewhat to a more controlled canter. He was still driving back to his office at Brookstone Police Station, currently just north of Benstown on the Great North Highway. Still with forty kilometres to go, he checked the time. To distract his thoughts onto something more constructive, he started to calculate what he had left to get done today.

He was the type of person who liked to get today's work done today, and would often work back late to complete tasks, just to make tomorrow easier. It was an infinite cycle, no matter how much he did today, tomorrow would always be just as busy, if not busier. No matter how determined he was to control his day, it always seemed to control him. Dick was determined today was going to end differently. He promised himself he would walk out the office door on time. His mood was uplifted by the prospect. It even managed to place him back into the present, as the music from the commercial radio started to register again.

He glanced at the police radio to check it was turned on. He had been so far away in his thoughts that he could not recall hearing anything from it for nearly an hour now. He reached down and turned its volume up.

The vivid images of the past were now replaced with the scenery surrounding him. Bushland, farming paddocks, and mine sites flashed by his window. He was even aware of the low rumble of road noise, as the tyres of his vehicle chewed away at the kilometres ahead.

Dick noticed that the steady stream of traffic flowing south, normal for this time of the day, was not there. He had clear vision to the next crest, a kilometre in the distance. There was not a single vehicle heading towards him. The road appeared to just end where its crest met the cloud dotted sky. One cloud appeared different to the others. It was much darker than the white clouds that turned ashen grey at their bases. The black cloud appeared to be growing, as it billowed further up into the sky above the crest.

At first, Dick was puzzled by the scene, but then assumed one of the coal mines that dotted the surrounding landscape must be blasting. It was not uncommon for the mining companies to close the highway for safety reasons when a blast was actually taking place nearby. He had noticed a ripple across his windscreen but put it down to the reflection of the sun. Dick now considered it must have been a shock wave from the mine blast.

Satisfied with his assumption, Dick started to slow as he approached the crest, expecting a line of traffic to be stopped just over the other side. Dick was right, and when he cleared the crest he found both north and south bound traffic at a standstill. The source of the billowing black cloud was far from being a mine blast, it was more like an Air Force jet had missed its bombing run at the military range and dropped its arsenal of explosives in the middle of the highway.

'My God,' were the only words to pass his lips to sum up what he saw.

It took Dick a few seconds to comprehend the carnage before him. Training then took over and he swung into action. He contacted police radio and informed them of the situation. He basically told the operator to get the emergency response phone book out, start at A and not to stop until he got to Z.

Dick activated his red and blue emergency warning lights as he drove on the wrong side of the road, past the line of stopped cars. Every so often he would give a blast of his siren as drivers started to get out of their cars and mingle on the roadway to gawk at the scene.

Arriving at the head of the queue, Dick parked his police vehicle and quickly climbed out. Just in front of him, a small sedan was partially blocking the south bound lane as it angled into the breakdown lane. The impact to the front of the car had been so great it tore the bonnet and engine bay clean off. What was left of the car was engulfed with fire.

Flames flared out through the smashed windows at Dick, as he tried to move closer.

The intense heat pushed him back. Dick's face felt like it had a blow torch held to it. He tried protecting his face with raised hands as he again tried to push closer. Again he was forced back from the searing heat and had to resign himself to the fact that he was not equipped to fight against such an intense beast. He considered the fire extinguisher he carried in his vehicle, but quickly disregarded its inadequacy.

Even at a distance of five metres, Dick struggled to hold his ground. His eyes searched inside the vehicle. Between bursts of red and orange, he could just make out the shape of a person behind the steering wheel. The flames that were consuming the car were also devouring the driver. The full outline of the driver was lost in the flames as Dick struggled to make out the person's head. The driver still appeared to be clutching the steering wheel with both hands. There was no movement by the driver to escape the inferno, and Dick could only assume that he had already burnt to death.

Above the roar of the fire, Dick could hear the hiss and sizzle of burning flesh. Then the pop, as moisture in the body was evaporated instantly as the skin blistered and bubbled. It was just like a steak had been placed onto a hot barbecue plate.

A mangled heap of steel and rubber, that was once the front of the car, was itself burning in bushland just off the highway. The surrounding trees and shrubs were ablaze. Sparks and burning embers were tossed high into the air and started further spot fires where they landed.

Dick circled the car from a distance. He considered that any passengers in the vehicle may have climbed out or been ejected, but instinct told him that no one could survive such a horrific impact. Even so, he started to search for anybody he could help. With his face still shielded by his hands, Dick rounded the rear of the car. Suddenly, one foot slipped out from under him. Dick fell to one knee, partially catching his fall. His hand went down onto the bitumen to prevent him falling further.

He felt something soft under his hand that was not at home on the hard bitumen. A stabbing pain then entered his palm as if stuck by a needle.

He steadied himself and looked at his hand as he raised it. There was no horror at what he saw. There was no shock or revulsion as Dick realised why he was unable to make out the driver's head in the car. Under his hand was the torn and bloodied meaty tissue of the driver's cheek. The sharp pain that Dick had felt was caused by a canine tooth. The cheek steak was still attached to one half of the driver's shattered bottom jaw, complete with incisors and molars.

Dick rose to his feet slowly. Once erect, he studied his palm. He felt nothing at all as he looked at his hand covered in blood. The hand did not even feel attached to him as he retrieved a handkerchief from his overalls and began to wipe the bloody residue from it.

His body was consumed by a calmness that he had felt many times before. The numbness that now consumed it also blocked out any sound from the scene around him. It was as if he had left his body and was now watching someone else go about a job. He finished wiping his hand and then casually returned the handkerchief to his pocket as if he had just blown his nose.

Dick saw no bodies lying on the roadway on the other side of the car. He turned around to look back at the cheek and jaw on the roadway. He scrutinised the surrounding roadway and now saw smaller portions of meaty tissue near it. A further three metres away, he noticed a larger piece. He had only taken one step towards it when he realised what it was. He now looked down upon it and the decapitated driver of the blazing car stared back at him. It was half a head, split down the middle. It was complete with hair, ear, eye, a portion of nose, and the rest of the mouth and jaw.

'That would have hurt,' Dick said voicelessly. He scoured the drainage ditch that lined the edge of the highway.
He searched the blackened areas of scrub that had now burnt themselves out. He found no other bodies.

The view up the highway towards Brookstone got no better as Dick now turned his attention there. The roadway was littered with vehicle debris. The bitumen was torn where metal had dug into it. The tattered roadway stretched for one-hundred metres, where another inferno blazed. A semi-trailer was ablaze and jack-knifed across both lanes.

A crowd of onlookers, who had left their own cars in the idle traffic, kept a safe distance away from the flames. 'Did anyone see the collision,' Dick yelled towards them in order to be heard over the flames.

No one replied. No one stepped forward, just heads shaking no.

'No one comes past my vehicle,' Dick again yelled at the crowd. He didn't want them contaminating the scene.

Satisfied there was nothing more he could do this end, Dick turned and started to jog towards the blazing truck, fully prepared to be greeted by another dead and burning body.

The fire that engulfed the truck was so intense that the bitumen around it had also caught on fire. The truck being so high, and with flames obscuring the cabin, Dick could not see if anyone was inside.

The big, solid prime mover showed only moderate damage from the impact with the car. It appeared that the outer edge of the truck's front bumper-bar had taken only a glancing blow. The full impact had been taken by the front right wheel and large external fuel tank. The tank had ruptured, spraying hundreds of litres of diesel over both vehicles. As volatile petrol lines from the car were torn from their fittings, a spark from grinding metal had ignited the highly flammable petrol in an explosive fireball. The oily diesel soon flared up and continued to burn as both vehicles parted and went on their separate, but fatal journeys. Spot fires littered the roadside bushland over the entire one-hundred metres that separated the two vehicles.

The truck obscured all vision to the other side of the highway. Dick was unable see the bank of traffic stopped in the southbound lane behind it as he gave the truck a wide berth to move to its other side. A crowd had gathered, as at the opposite end of the carnage. The difference was that this crowd was not so much watching the burning rig, but huddled around a man sitting on the roadway and propped against the side of the first car in the queue.

The truck driver had escaped his fiery tomb with only a few bruises and singed whiskers. Shock was now his main injury. Several other motorists knelt beside him. One had even wrapped him in a space blanket from a first aid kit he carried in his car.

'Is this the truck driver?' Dick asked.

'Yeah, it's a miracle he's alive,' came the man's reply.

Dick was looking at the shaking truck driver when he asked, 'Was there anyone else in the truck?' The truck driver just stared past Dick vacantly as if he was not even there.

'He told me it was just him in the truck,' the other man replied. 'A few of the other blokes had a look around. They didn't find anyone else.'

Dick noticed two cars were parked facing in the opposite direction to the queue of cars pointing south.

'Did any of you see the collision?' asked Dick towards the crowd.

Two men at the front put their hands up like students in a classroom. 'We did,' one of them said hesitantly. 'We were following directly behind the truck. He didn't have a chance. The car just veered straight into him.'

'…and veered late,' the second witness added.

Dick had the two witnesses give him their driver's licences.

He did not want them leaving the scene without obtaining their details. 'Don't go anywhere,' Dick told the two witnesses. 'We'll get statements from you shortly.'

The two witnesses did not protest and seemed happy to help out.

'Same with you two,' Dick said towards the men comforting the truck driver.

'We're not going to leave our mate here,' one said, already having bonded to the man in a way that only adversity can.

'An ambulance shouldn't be too far away,' Dick said to the group. 'I'm heading back down the other end. More police and the fire brigade should be here shortly.' Dick turned and walked several paces before being stopped by a question.

'How did the others fair down that end?'

Dick turned to face the first witness who had spoken, and just shook his head. He then started to jog back towards his police vehicle to update police radio of the situation.

3.30PM

Rowdy could not help but ask the dumb question as he continued to hold the head of a dead man. 'How is he?'

The ambulance officer, who had climbed inside the car from the passenger side, had just finished examining Lindsay and without a hint of emotion to his words replied, 'He is currently displaying symptoms which are not conducive to life.'

The ambulance officer extracted himself from the vehicle, then, in either hand picked up his medical kit and oxy reviver bottle he had left outside the passenger door. His work was done here. He walked towards Lynda, still nestled in Mel's arms, quietly sobbing.

The news from the ambulance officer that confirmed Lindsay's death initially confused Rowdy. He had no idea what to do next. He knew he could let go of Lindsay's head but did not want to. This only managed to confuse him more, because emotionally, he actually felt nothing. He failed to understand the bond that had developed between himself and the man he held. He now focused his attention towards Lynda who had been watching him intently. She was still waiting for the news that her husband was OK and going to live. Rowdy removed his hands and allowed the blood sodden jumper to drop into Lindsay's lap. His skull immediately parted again to reveal its slurry of contents.

Rowdy slowly withdrew his crimson gloved hands back out through the window. The certainty of Lindsay's death now showed heavily on his face and tore at his soul. Lynda's reaction was immediate. The grief of losing her husband was released with the force of a dam wall breaching. Mel was caught unaware. Lynda, unable to support her own weight collapsed through the comforting woman's arms to the ground. Her whole body shook as she babbled in utter distress, 'He only wanted a meat pie.'

As Rowdy watched the distraught woman, all he could do was chastise himself. How could he be so insensitive to feel no compassion towards her? He felt no urge to comfort her. He just wanted to leave, but something inside him prevented it.

Mel sat on the ground with her arms once more wrapped around Lynda. Mel rocked her as one would when soothing a child. The ambulance officer knelt on one knee beside them and started to unravel the oxygen mask attached to the cylinder that he placed on the bitumen next to them.

A noise from inside the car startled Rowdy. He soon recognised the trumpeting tune as the Mexican Hat Dance. It was a mobile phone ring tone, which Rowdy traced to a bulge in Lindsay's trouser pocket. His first reaction was to answer the phone, and opened the driver's door, but quickly convinced himself that no good could possibly come from doing that. The song stopped playing as abruptly as it had started and the phone went to message bank.

Rowdy was about to close the door again when he caught a glimpse of a dark, elongated object in the floor well beside the driver's seat. The metal bar had fallen between the door and seat after piercing through Lindsay's head. The bar was mostly covered in dull, powdery, surface rust, except for one end, which appeared to shine. The dark shimmering gloss travelled along the shaft for a short distance. Rowdy leaned down to inspect it closely. The lustre was caused by a smearing of blood. The reality that he was looking at the object responsible for Lindsay's death now struck him. He refrained from picking up the bar and left it undisturbed for later scientific examination, to assist in determining where it came from, and who it belonged to.

After removing his gloves, Rowdy reached into his pocket and removed his own mobile phone. He dialled his wife.

'Hi Em,' he said overly cheerful.

'What's wrong,' Emma suspiciously enquired as she stopped folding the washing, the cordless phone propped on an ear with her shoulder.

Rowdy continued to feign a cheery persona. 'Nothing's wrong. I'm a bit tied up, that's all.'

Emma took the phone in her hand and in a worried voice asked, 'Where are the kids?'

'That's why I'm calling,' he answered nervously, unsure how his wife was going to handle the news. 'They're still at school. I'm not going to be able to pick them up. Can you duck into town and get them?'

Emma's first reaction was annoyance. Her children would be late for their dentist appointment. Her annoyance quickly subsided though. She knew Rowdy was the type of man who would put himself out before he shirked on his word.

'That's no problem,' replied Emma in a composed voice that belied her concern for her husband. 'I'll ring and cancel my hair appointment.'

'Thanks Em. I'm really sorry, but there's been another accident and I can't get away,' he replied, without going into any details. Emma could sense in his voice that there was something terribly wrong. She knew her husband rarely went into great detail about his work, but she could well imagine what things must be like. With Rowdy, an accident meant anything from a small dent to a multiple fatality.

'Just look after yourself,' Emma said with concern.

'I'm fine,' was Rowdy's expected reply. 'You better give the dentist a quick ring and let them know you might be a bit late.'

Emma's voice was soothing, 'Don't worry. I'll take care of it.'

'Thanks again Em. I'll meet you later on at the kids' school play.'

He disconnected the call. He looked back at the horror of Lindsay's disfigured head. He watched as the ambulance staff went about their work, placing Lynda onto a gurney and wheeling her towards the rear of the ambulance with its high-swing tailgate open. The fire brigade were arriving and preparing their hoses.

'How lucky am I,' Rowdy's inner voice said as he counted his blessings. It could just as easily have been him sitting in that car, caught in the wrong place at the wrong moment in time. To top it all off, he considered how fortunate he was to be married to such a loving, considerate, and compassionate woman as Emma. His sombre mood brightened a little as he replaced the scene before his eyes with the attractive and elegant portrait of his wife.

The hanging victim's waist was just below Ricky's head. The man was dressed in faded, blue jeans, and flannelette shirt with the sleeves rolled up. Ricky reached up and patted down the dead man's waist and legs. In a front pocket he located a bundle of keys. The largest was obviously a car key. Ricky reached over to the driver's door of the car and found it locked. Tombstone was on the passenger side and was met with the same result when he lifted the door handle.

'These might help,' said Ricky, tossing the keys over the roof.

Tombstone raised a large hand in front of his face and caught the keys. 'Why would you lock your car to commit suicide?' he asked, rubbing his jaw in contemplation.

'I don't know,' shrugged Ricky, without giving the question much thought. 'I still haven't answered the question of why you would commit suicide in the first place.'

Tombstone inserted the key, and with a quarter turn, all the locking mechanisms clunked open.

'Makes you wonder what goes through a person's mind, though, doesn't it?' said Tombstone, continuing to ponder on the reason. The constant questioning of things is what made Tombstone such an effective policeman. Frustratingly, most questions could not be given a rational answer.

'Maybe he just didn't want someone stealing his car,' offered Ricky while removing a wallet from the man's rear pocket.

He inspected the wallet's contents and found thirty dollars along with some loose change and the man's driver's licence. Behind the inner front clear plastic display was a family photograph. It depicted a husband and wife each nursing a young child. Both children would have been under five years of age. The faces in the portrait were all smiles.

Ricky took a step back and raised the open wallet into the air. He lifted the wallet to his line of sight, just below the victim's angled and swollen head. He compared the two images.

'Not your most photogenic angle mate, but I can see the similarities,' said Ricky to the deceased, and satisfied himself that it was the same person as in the photo.

Tombstone had half his body buried inside the small four-wheel-drive when he heard Ricky's muffled voice. He extracted himself and looked back over the roof at Ricky. 'You say something?'

'Just having a conversation with my new mate here,' replied Ricky.

Tombstone could see Ricky holding the open wallet. 'Who have we got?' he quizzed.

Ricky removed the licence and said, 'We have one Reginald Arthur Boyd and he's a local Chifley boy according to his address.'

Tombstone walked around the vehicle and took the licence from Ricky. 'I'll just run a check on the car's registration,' he said and walked over to the police truck.

Ricky placed the wallet onto the bonnet of the four-wheel-drive and continued to search the deceased. Other than a wrist watch, he found no other property. He then opened the rear passenger door next to the dangling legs. Ricky stood on the sill and rotated the body. He could not locate any blood stains or damage to clothing which may have indicated wounds of some kind.

Tombstone returned and tossed the driver's licence onto the bonnet, next to the wallet. He retrieved the bundle of keys from his pocket and placed them on top of the victim's wallet.

'The car belongs to him,' said Tombstone. 'The bushwalker who located him is now at the station making a statement.'

'Is there an ETA for the body snatchers?' asked Ricky.

'They'll be here by four-o'clock,' replied Tombstone. 'We'll just do a quick search of the surrounding bushland in the meantime.'

'Is there anything out of place in the car?' Ricky asked his offsider.

'Only a suicide note left on the seat,' said Tombstone as he walked around to open a door. 'Everything else gives the impression it's just an ordinary family car.'

Leaning inside the driver's door, Tombstone read from the handwritten note.

> *'My amazing Jules,*
> *Please don't blame yourself for this. It is completely my fault for what I have done. I try as hard as I can but I continually fail. Everything is just falling apart around me. I haven't done this to hurt you or the kids. I love you all so much but if I continue on the way I am I will only cause you all pain. You will find happiness without me. I am no fun for anyone. I hate myself, no one else.*
> *I'm sorry. Please forgive me   Reggie.'*

'You would have thought he could have added a postscript,' Ricky said when Tombstone finished reading.

Tombstone gave a quizzical look. 'And what would that be?' he asked.

'Thanks to the poor coppers who have to clean up my mess,' said Ricky, with a hint of anger in his voice caused by the man's selfish act. His displeasure for the man only grew when he considered the young family that he had given up on.

'Don't take it personally Ricky,' Tombstone said with a straight face. 'By the look of him, I don't think he cares.'

The two officers started their search of the surrounding bushland at the same point, they headed off in opposite directions. They would then overlap and search the half that the other had just completed, just to be thorough.

Dick stood at the rear of his police vehicle, having updated the radio operator of the situation. Dick's fingerprint and DNA work could often be a messy one, so he always carried a twenty litre container of water with a tap fitted. He stood under the raised tailgate and washed the blood stains off his hand. A liberal amount of antibacterial foam was then worked into them. He felt no need to rush. There was nothing that he could do.

He now heard the faint sound of sirens in the distant. Their pitch increased rapidly as the emergency vehicles approached at high speed. Dick casually walked down to the small car that was still burning but not with the same intensity as before. He positioned himself to direct the emergency response vehicles.

The first to appear was the local Benstown General Duties truck crew. Dick stood in line with the partial head and other body parts that littered the roadway. He pointed to his right for the police vehicle to move over.

The last thing he wanted was to see a head stuck onto the tyre of the police truck, flopping over and over.

'Hi Dick,' greeted the driver of the police truck as he stopped beside him. 'Nice little party you have here. Thanks for the invitation.'

'Wouldn't want you boys missing all the fun,' said Dick in good humour that disguised his true feelings. 'Now make yourself useful and go down the other end to that truck. The driver is out and okay. Just drive down the breakdown lane. There's some physical evidence on the road I want to preserve.'

Dick saw no point in telling the two officers in the truck about the slice of head and other fragments. The less who saw it, the better.

'What do you want to do about this traffic?' asked the junior officer.

'Nothing at the moment,' Dick replied. 'We'll let the fire personnel get these flames under control first before we look at getting traffic flowing again. They get upset when cars drive over their hoses.'

Dick then handed the driver of the police truck the two driver's licences he took from the witnesses. 'Grab statements off these two blokes while you're down there,' directed Dick.

The police truck roared off just as an ambulance approached from behind. Dick stopped it and explained about the truck driver and directed them down the breakdown lane as well.

At last two fire tankers arrived. Their wailing sirens were a vast contrast to the sluggish speed at which they approached, burdened down by their heavy load of water and equipment.

Dick spoke with the Fire Captain. 'Where do you want to start?' he asked the fire chief.

The Fire Captain quickly appraised the scene.

'We'll get this scrub fire under control first, before it turns into a raging bushfire. There's another two tankers close behind. I'll have them make a start on the vehicles.'

Dick quickly explained about the incinerated body inside the car so the Captain could warn his men. He also appraised him about the body parts as they would be required to work close to them.

Dick could do nothing else as the fire crews sprang into action. The loud humming of water pumps soon mixed with the crackle of flames.

4PM

'What now?' Ricky asked, finding only rabbit holes and ant nests in their search of the surrounding bushland.

A mischievous look appeared on Tombstone's face. 'We toss the coin,' he said with a broad grin, then looked up at the hanging victim.

'Why are we tossing a coin?' asked a confused Ricky.

Tombstone prolonged Ricky's bewilderment. 'Well there isn't much else left to do here.'

Ricky knew his partner was setting him up for something, so he started to play the game. After all, Tombstone was right. Until the funeral contractors arrived, there was little else to do.

'It's been a long day Tombstone; you're not as young as you used to be so why don't you just take a nice rest in the police truck.'

Tombstone absorbed the insult without flinching. 'But if we don't toss the coin, I'll have to pull rank on you.'

'Pull rank,' retorted Ricky. 'So it's not just bad luck that I get all the shitty jobs?'

'This could be your lucky day, though, if we toss the coin,' Tombstone replied genuinely. 'At least you would have a fifty-fifty chance of not getting the next shitty job.'

Ricky was wary of the big old senior constable. 'Now you're just getting my hopes up so you can shatter them. You'll take great delight in watching me fall.'

'Actually,' Tombstone said, then turned and looked up at the dead man swinging in the breeze. 'I was counting on someone else taking the fall.'

Ricky paused as he looked at the dead man and contemplated Tombstone's words.

'So you're talking about getting this bloke down?' he said, as the realisation struck him.

'That's right,' confirmed Tombstone with a satisfied smile.

'I thought we would just cut him down,' Ricky said, somewhat surprised that there was another option.

'Cutting him down will be part of it,' explained Tombstone. 'But we just can't let him fall to the ground.'

'He's dead,' Ricky exclaimed. 'He's not going to complain.'

Tombstone's expression turned serious for a moment when he replied, 'But his family might.'

Ricky made a point of looking over each shoulder before he said, 'But they're not here. How will they know?'

'They'll know when they get a copy of the Coroner's Report which will list his broken limbs or dislocated hips, with the notation that those injuries were inflicted by police,' explained Tombstone.

Ricky felt stupid he had not considered these consequences. More importantly he felt embarrassed for not treating the deceased with appropriate respect. Joking about the situation was one thing. Causing further harm to the deceased and family was inexcusable.

'Cheer up, Ricky,' said Tombstone as if reading his mind. 'Chalk it all up to experience.'

Ricky smiled at Tombstone. 'You're not only old, but wise too,' he said to lighten his mood.

'Comes with the age and experience son,' Tombstone said, taking the remark as a compliment. 'Now back to the important issue, the coin toss.'

'Okay, fill me in,' said Ricky.

'To prevent this poor sod falling like a sack of potatoes, we need a catcher,' Tombstone now explained.

'And I'm the catcher,' Ricky said, finishing Tombstone's sentence for him.

'Due to your rank in the food chain, the answer would normally be yes,' replied Tombstone. 'But today, I'm going to give you a chance to be the cutter.'

'The coin toss,' Ricky now said with clarity.

With a wink and click of the tongue, Tombstone said, 'That's right.'

Ricky held out his hand and gave Tombstone a suspicious look. 'Show me the coin first,' he said.

'I'm hurt,' said Tombstone and clutched a hand to his chest as if it had just been pierced by an arrow. 'To think you don't trust me.'

Ricky continued to hold out his hand and now motioned his fingers to add meaning to his words, 'Come on, the coin.'

Tombstone removed a coin from his fob pocket and placed it into Ricky's open palm. Ricky jiggled his hand slightly as if it was a set of scales measuring the weight. He then held it by the edge, between his thumb and index finger, to examine both sides closely. Ricky still had his suspicions and cast Tombstone a wary eye.

'Tell you what. To be impartial, let's use one of his,' said Ricky, and thumbed in the direction of the deceased.

Tombstone laughed at Ricky's paranoia. 'If that'll make you feel better, fine.'

Ricky took the wallet off the bonnet of the car and removed a fifty cent piece from the coin pouch.

'I'll even let you toss the coin,' Tombstone now said to alleviate any further mistrust, adding, 'Do you want our friend here to call?'

'If he does, I'll have to shoot him,' Ricky said with his hand on his revolver. 'How will that look on the Coroner's Report?'

Ricky tossed the coin high into the air. 'Heads,' he called. The coin flickered in the tree filtered sunlight as it reached the peak of its arc, then fell to the ground with a dull thud. A small bloom of dust rose as the coin partially buried itself into the powdery soil. Both men stooped forward.

One began a laugh that started deep down in his belly, then developed into convulsions as his entire body began to shake. The other just starred at the image of a kangaroo and emu holding a shield.

Tombstone had to wipe tears of laughter from his eyes as he blurringly watched Ricky delicately pick up the coin and turn it over to double check the bust of the Queen was actually on the coin.

'Looks like Her Majesty has decided it's not your lucky day after all,' Tombstone managed to say as his laughter abated.

'Shit,' Ricky cursed and placed the coin back in the wallet. 'I'll never salute her again.'

The low rumble of tyres on gravel was now heard approaching the clearing. The white funeral director's van appeared, rocking as it traversed the potholed track.

'Good-day again, gentlemen,' Tombstone cheerily said to the short and tall man as they exited their van. Their frail features still indicating they had not had a descent feed since their last encounter, earlier that morning.

The two men set about removing a gurney from the van and then parked it beside the hanging victim. Tombstone briefly explained his plan of attack to safely lower the body.

Ricky faced the deceased and nestled the side of the dead man's waist between his head and shoulder. He wrapped his arms around the top half of the man's legs like a footballer going into a tackle. Ricky braced himself to take the dead weight.

'Are you ready?' asked Tombstone, who was standing at the front of the four-wheel-drive. He placed the blade of his pocket knife against the rope where it tied onto the bull bar.

'Whenever you're ready,' came Ricky's muffled reply and pulled the dead man tighter into his cheek.

The two spindly funeral assistants grasped the rope above where Tombstone began to slice in a sawing action, not confident the two men were going to be of much help to slowly lower the body. Considering their skeletal frames, Tombstone had visions of them being yanked over the car when the rope was severed.

He was proven wrong. With Ricky supporting the body, the two funeral assistants managed to lower the body in a controlled, steady fashion. Ricky moved sideways towards the gurney. The deceased was lowered onto the bed and Ricky released his tackle hold to then push the upper torso of the man by the shoulders, back onto the bed. The two funeral staff continued to feed out the rope until the man's body lay flat on the trolley. Tombstone lifted the man's legs onto the gurney.

'Job well done,' Tombstone congratulated everyone.

Dick walked up to the firemen as they were shutting down their hoses. The flames that engulfed the small car were extinguished. The thick smoke that had bloomed into the sky was now reduced to fine slivers, as it snaked its way up out of the car's windows that had shattered out from the intense heat. The duco had blistered off, stripping the car back to bare metal which was now scorched black, and already showed signs of oxidisation as patches of rust-brown appeared.

The steel rims of the rear wheels sat tireless in the melted roadway. Clumps of molten rubber pooled around them, with strands of their inner steel belts exposed.

Police have a statutory authority to take charge of all emergencies. However, if that emergency involved fire, then the Fire Brigade took charge until the fire was extinguished.

'Can I approach the vehicle, guys?' said Dick, asking permission as he drew near the group of firemen from behind.

'All yours again,' confirmed the leader of the group and relinquished control of the scene back to Dick.

'I wouldn't touch any of the metal just yet. It could still be pretty hot,' he added as a warning.

Dick passed through the line of firemen. 'Just want to check how many bodies we have,' he said. Inside the car was just a shell. All the seats had been reduced to their metal frames and springs. What plastic mouldings failed to melt to the floor, formed abstract artworks as they sagged into molten shapes.

Dick found only the headless driver inside the vehicle. He again felt no repulsion at what he saw. He turned and faced the firemen who crept forward, still on standby with their hoses trained on the car.

'I don't want you blokes any closer,' Dick snapped firmly, and out of character.

Dick now felt something that he had never felt before. He was no longer concerned with protecting and preserving the scene, but more interested in protecting others from the scene. Even though he felt no emotional connection to the horrific sight of the charred driver, he instinctively knew that it could be traumatising to others. He was now determined to prevent as many people as possible from seeing the remains, both in the vehicle, and on the roadway.

Anger, that Dick struggled to control, for some reason swelled within him. 'Get me two tarps,' he again snapped at the firemen.

Refusing assistance from the fire personnel, Dick spread one tarp over the slice of head and other human tissue that littered the road. He then struggled with the second to heave its weight up and over the car.

'It's times like this you need some privacy my friend,' Dick said to the headless man as he disappeared from view.

The driver was a blackened, charred mess. Under the old classification, he had sustained fifth and sixth degree burns. His synthetic clothing melted into him as all skin and subcutaneous tissues were destroyed to expose muscle. In areas such as his arms, where the depth of tissue was not as great, the fire had burnt through to expose bone. 'There would be no fingerprinting this body,' Dick thought to himself as he secured the canvass. Dick even managed to string up some blue and white checked police tape around the car and the tarp laid out on the road, creating a physical barrier as well as visual.

Two more police vehicles now arrived on scene. One contained Inspector Rob Cooley, a Duty Officer from the Coal Valley Local Area Command. The other contained two more General Duty police.

'Hi boss,' Dick said as the Inspector approached.

'What have you got under your handy work here, Dick?' the Inspector enquired, indicating towards the tarps and police tape.

Dick informed the Duty Officer and the other two constables of the gruesome scene. He also updated them on the truck situation at the other end, which now had its flames extinguished.

Inspector Cooley was now the senior ranking officer on scene and automatically assumed command. Dick had to show some diplomacy as he suggested to his boss what he would like done next.

'Boss, if you would like to liaise with the Fire Captain, I'd like to get some of this traffic moving down this northern breakdown lane,' proposed Dick.

The scrub fire now appeared under control, but to ensure no toes were stepped on, Dick wanted the Fire Captain's approval. The safety of all personnel working at the scene was still a major consideration and Dick did not want anyone run over once the traffic started to move again.

'Good idea,' Inspector Cooley replied. 'Unfortunately there is nowhere to detour traffic around this section of the highway.'

The breakdown lane was the best they could do for a single lane. At least they would start the traffic flowing as they alternated between north and south.

'Do you know how far the Crash Investigation Unit is away?' Dick asked the Inspector.

The Inspector shook his head. 'They're tied up with another accident,' he said without expanding. 'The Crime Scene Unit will be attending instead. Fortunately, Ben Ford was passing through the area and isn't too far away.'

Dick knew Senior Constable Ben Ford and highly respected him as a Crime Scene Investigator. He knew the accident scene would be in good hands.

He noticed one of the young General Duty officers bend down and pass under the police tape. 'Where are you going?' Dick shouted with instant aggression towards the young officer.

The officer kept walking towards the tarp that covered the roadway and said, 'I'm just going to have a look under here.'

'No you're not,' said Dick sharply, continuing with his aggressive tone. 'Get your arse out of there.' Dick started to walk purposefully towards the young officer who could now see his wide eyed and fiery expression.

The young officer persisted, 'I'm not going to touch anything, just take a look.'

Becoming more enraged, Dick's hands clenched tightly into fists. He was just about to let fly with a verbal spray threatening physical harm towards the officer when Inspector Cooley stepped in and voiced loudly, 'Do as you're told, son.'

The young officer returned to near his vehicle, giving Dick a wide berth.

Inspector Cooley knew that Dick's reaction was totally out of character. In all the years that he had known him, he had never seen him display an ounce of aggression. In fact, he was one of the quietest and most placid people he had ever met.

'You alright?' Cooley asked when Dick returned.

Dick had a confused look. 'Yeah, why wouldn't I be?' he said calmly.

The Inspector did not probe any further. He spoke with the Fire Captain and within minutes one lane of traffic was moving slowly along the breakdown lane as a police officer at either end performed point duty.

A Forensic Services van arrived soon afterwards. Dick gave Senior Constable Ben Ford a concise overview of the scene.

Rowdy was just returning the mobile phone to his pocket after speaking with his wife. He swung around as a voice came from behind him. 'You pick a fine time to ring and order pizza.'

Bryan approached Rowdy while Baz was still getting out of his highway car. Rowdy had not heard or seen them arrive. He now relaxed and replied to his long time work colleague. 'If I had known you were coming, I would have super-sized it.'

Bryan ignored the innuendo directed at his girth and said, 'I heard on the radio you were in a spot of bother so I've come to bail you out… again.' He looked over at Lindsay's body in the car. 'Who's your friend?'

'Don't know,' replied Rowdy, 'but unlike Bill Clinton, I think I've just had an intimate relationship with him.'

Bryan again looked at the disfigured man, this time with some concern on his face. 'I'm disappointed in you Rowdy,' he said in mock seriousness. 'He's not even very attractive.'

The Mexican Hat Dance again trumpeted from the mobile phone in Lindsay's pocket. Both men turned in unison towards the sound.

'It's just his mobile phone,' explained Rowdy.

Baz now joined them and entered the light hearted conversation when he said, 'That gives new meaning to being temporarily unavailable. Please leave a message, now doesn't it?' and peered at Lindsay.

Rowdy turned serious and explained the situation to his colleagues. The mystery of the metal bar was still to be solved. He started to organise the investigation.

'You two speak with that lady over there,' said Rowdy and pointed towards Mel. 'If she witnessed what happened, get a statement from her.'

The local Bowen fire tanker now arrived. Rowdy approached the Fire Captain and briefed him. He then issued instructions for a tarp to be placed over the vehicle. Fortunately the highway was not blocked or obstructed in any way, but motorists had slowed considerably on seeing all the flashing lights of the emergency vehicles. They were all rubber necking, keen to see what was happening. The sooner Lindsay's grotesque body could be covered, the better.

Rowdy neared the rear of the ambulance. He was dreading having to speak with the woman who was now sitting up on the bed.

'Can I speak with her?' he asked the ambulance officer who was sitting beside her, more for comfort than medical assistance.

'Sure thing,' the officer replied. 'Her heart rate and blood pressure are up a bit so we're going to take her to hospital for observation. Just make it brief.'

Rowdy climbed into the rear of the ambulance and sat opposite Lynda. He first recorded her details and those of her husband. He asked what happened and Lynda recounted the minutes before her life, and husband's head, shattered. She soon became agitated as she spoke of the shattering windscreen. Rowdy pushed her no further. There would be plenty of time later to take a more formal statement.

Bryan and Baz had finished interviewing Mel and compared notes with Rowdy.

'Both women mention a passing truck,' Rowdy said in contemplation. 'The obvious conclusion is that the bar has fallen from this passing truck.'

'Or,' Bryan added, 'the bar was already on the road and has been tossed up by the truck driving over it.'

'What about the safety-cam?' Baz added to the conversation, wide eyed with inspiration.

The State Traffic Authority operates a heavy vehicle monitoring system known as Safe-T-Cam. It was an automated digital camera system that recorded heavy vehicle number plates at twenty-four locations around the state. The initiative was designed to improve road safety by reducing truck crashes due to speed and fatigue. It also enforces vehicle registration offences.

'Of course!' Rowdy exclaimed. 'There's a safety-cam monitoring site a kilometre up the highway. Baz, you're brilliant, regardless of what everyone else says.'

Baz beamed with pride at being able to make a contribution to the investigation.

'Get on the radio,' Rowdy now instructed Baz. 'Have them contact the Traffic Authority to get whoever works that safety-cam system to pull every detail and photo of every truck that has passed through at the time of the collision, and fifteen minutes either side.'

There was no urgency to do this as the truck was now long gone from the area. Rowdy just knew from experience, though, that the sooner leads were followed up, the greater chance of success. Baz, overcome with enthusiasm, raced off towards his highway car.

'The only other time I've seen him move that fast is when he's chasing women,' Bryan joked.

Rowdy pointed down the highway towards Bowen. 'The Crash Investigation boys have moved fast too,' he said to Bryan as he spotted the Kingstown based unit speeding towards them.

Bryan studied the approaching police vehicle, but his attention was soon drawn to the vehicle travelling closely behind it at a matching speed.

'But look who's taking a free ride on his coat tails,' Bryan now said as he made out the vehicle of a regional television media crew.

4.30PM

Dick assisted the Crime Scene officer gather his necessary tools from the rear of the forensic van. Senior Constable Ben Ford sat on the rear bumper reloading a fresh roll of film into his camera. The thigh pocket of his overalls bulged, stuffed with spare rolls.

He pulled open a number of drawers lining one side of the van, searching for the evidence bags that would be required to collect the slice of head and other facial parts.

'Where do you keep your plastic bags, Ben?' Dick asked in defeat.

'Top far left,' said Ben without looking up from what he was doing.

Dick had already pulled open another wrong draw. 'I assume you won't need this,' he said and presented a long glass thermometer for Ben to see.

The rectal thermometer was often used on corpses to record their core body temperature. The reading would then assist in establishing a time of death.

'Not unless you need to check if he's well done,' replied Ben lightly.

'I think we can safely say he's over done,' said Dick and placed the thermometer away.

Ben handed Dick a clipboard. 'You can be my scribe, while I measure and photograph.'

The accident scene was now under the capable command of the Duty Officer and other police. Traffic was flowing slowly past by alternating the directions of travel along the breakdown lane.

It was apparent that the deceased driver of the car was at fault when he crossed the centre line, into the oncoming truck. No criminal action could be taken as the driver had already paid the ultimate price for his actions, which exceeded what any Court in the land could impose. All that could be done now was record the scene for the Coroner and try to establish why the headless driver did what he did.

Even though the small car had been reduced to a burnt-out shell, it would still be impounded for mechanical examination to determine if mechanical or structural failure had contributed. Autopsy results would establish if the driver was affected by alcohol or other drugs, as well as rule out heart attack or other medical conditions which may shine light onto why the driver swerved into the path of a semi-trailer. The driver's last known movements leading up to the collision would also be investigated to take into account fatigue as a cause. Even the possibility of suicide would be considered.

Whatever the cause, Dick was now happy to be recording the scene for evidentiary purposes, something that his methodical nature made him good at. The scale of this scene was the only thing that differed from his day to day fingerprint and DNA work. In many ways, the dead were easier to deal with than the hostile or drunken, obnoxious clients that police dealt with on a daily basis.

Dick and Ben worked well together, starting at the car and decapitated body it contained, then working along the one-hundred metres of highway towards the truck. Dick was recording all the distances with an electronic measuring wheel as they walked. The pair stopped every few metres to record and take photographs of the damaged road pavement or an item from one of the vehicles.

About halfway towards the truck, Ben had to stand in the breakdown lane, which was now being used as a traffic lane, in order to achieve the right angle for one of his photos. Dick raised a hand to signal the vehicles approaching to stop.

To emphasis the point, he walked into the centre of the breakdown lane, in front of the vehicle he wanted the line of traffic to stop behind.

Rather than stop a safe distance from Dick, the driver of the first car edged forward to within millimetres of Dick before stopping. The driver leaned an elbow through his open window, followed by his head. 'Fuck me mate,' said the driver as he vented his frustration at being held up again onto Dick. 'I've been waiting half an hour already.

Dick told himself to remain calm and glanced at Ben who had already started to take his photos. 'Sorry mate, we're not going to be long.' Dick replied as he turned back towards the driver.

The driver continued to verbalise his annoyance towards Dick.

'Hurry the fuck up,' the driver yelled, followed by a blast of his car horn. 'Some of us hard workers have got lives to get on with you know.'

Dick managed to hold his tongue as his own anger threatened to vent from his lips. He was determined, though, not to reduce himself to the same level as the foul mouthed, hostile, and impatient driver. The driver again leant on the car's horn.

Ben could hear the one-sided exchange. He bent down on one knee in the middle of the breakdown lane and reached into his thigh pocket for a fresh role of film. 'I won't be long, Dick,' Ben called out. 'I just have to change a roll of film.'

The driver saw what was happening and became infuriated. He began to bombard Dick with a machine gun fire of expletives. The anger inside Dick was now replaced with amusement. He laughed inwardly as he watched the driver froth at the mouth and wave his arms to animate his words.

Ben removed the half used role of film and loaded a fresh one into his camera. He then pretended to take some more shots, just to prolong the driver's wait further.

'All done,' Ben shouted towards Dick then walked out of the breakdown lane.

Dick took several steps to the side of the stopped car and casually waved it on. Its driver revved the engine while ramming the manual gear shift into first and dropped the clutch. All he succeeded in doing was kangaroo hop several metres then stall the motor.

Flustered with embarrassment, the driver fumbled to restart the car, and then crunched the gearbox into first after forgetting to push in the clutch. He stalled for a second time. The cars waiting patiently behind now sounded their horns, directed more in amusement towards the antics of the driver in front than their own frustration. The musical tune of car horns became infectious with more and more drivers joining in until the lead driver finally got his car moving.

Dick and Ben both stared at the driver with comical looks plastered across their faces. His offensive outbursts had now been reduced to mumbles under his breath as he passed the two officers without making eye contact.

Most of the proceeding drivers gave a thumbs up or friendly wave as they passed the officers. The car directly behind the agitated driver had heard and witnessed the goings on and hollered as he passed, 'Good work guys.'

'Who said this job isn't fun,' said Dick as he began to walk the measuring wheel in the direction of the truck again.

The Crash Investigation officer busied himself recording and photographing the scene after being given a briefing by Rowdy.

The ambulance had left with Lynda on board. Rowdy had told Mel she was free to go home, but she was reluctant to leave for some reason.

Perhaps she was in the same position as Rowdy and felt a connection with the event and could not leave until everything was finished. She remained out of the way, quietly watching.

A television cameraman was busy taking footage of the scene as well. He focused his shoulder mounted camera on the Crash Investigation officer as he placed the metal object into an evidence bag. Even though the cameraman had taken footage of the car without the tarp covering Lindsay's body, Rowdy knew that they would only show those angles on the six o'clock news that did not reveal Lindsay's grotesque appearance. Just to be sure, though, Rowdy approached the reporter, who accompanied the cameraman, and reinforced the point.

The reporter, with notebook and pen in hand, asked Rowdy what happened. Rowdy was aware that all media units had police radio scanners, so the reporter would already have a good idea. Even so, he willingly obliged to an interview. It was better to keep a good working relationship with the media than not. Particularly in this case, where the media could help to assist find out if a truck was involved.

Following the interview, the cameraman continued to take further footage of the scene, this time of the fire brigade personnel, who were standing by with their hoses trained on Lindsay's car. Satisfied that they had sufficient footage to edit together a thirty second news segment, the media crew began to pack up. They had a deadline to meet. Rowdy watched until they drove out of sight. He knew they were equipped with highly sensitive directional microphones and would often park hundreds of metres away to try and pick up conversations at the scene. They would hope to glean additional information from idle chit chat amongst the emergency workers, information that would not normally be directly shared with them.

All anyone could do now is wait for the Crash Investigation officer to finish his work.

The relative silence of the scene was broken as a trumpet started to play the Mexican Hat Dance again. Although muted in Lindsay's pocket, the sound spread over the area and brought a festive air to the sombre scene.

Bryan attempted a quick Mexican tap dance, followed by an 'Olay.' The sight of a rather overweight police officer trying to pull off an act that required more co-ordination than he possessed, was not met with applause.

'You're a tough audience,' said Bryan, lowering his arms from above his head. He then hitched his gun belt and trousers up.

Bryan and Baz would finish at eight. Rowdy should have finished at three-thirty, so it made sense that he should hand the scene over to his two colleagues and leave. But, like Mel, Rowdy felt connected. He would see it through until the end.

A nondescript white van pulled up at the scene without making a noise to announce its arrival. Two men got out from either side of the van and approached Rowdy and Bryan.

'Looks like the body snatchers are circling,' Bryan said to Rowdy as he spotted the funeral contractors.

One of the contractors produced an information and security tag for Rowdy to complete. The tag system alleviated the need for police to attend the morgue and identify bodies. Rowdy was often resistant to change, but this was one modification to a system that he embraced. The less time spent at the morgue the better, as far as he was concerned.

'There's something about those guys I just don't like,' Bryan said, now the two funeral contractors had returned to wait in their van.

'It's only a problem if they're coming for you,' replied Rowdy philosophically.

Bryan continued to eyeball the two men. 'That's just it, you never know do you?'

Ricky changed down through the gears of the compact four-wheel-drive as he slowed to turn into the rear compound of Chifley Police Station. He followed close behind the police truck driven by Tombstone on their return from the suicide scene.

It had been an eerie trip for Ricky as he drove the hanging victim's vehicle out of the bush. He couldn't quite put his finger on the feeling he felt. It was somewhere between bizarre and that dirty feeling that always surrounds death.

Ricky had been studying the inside of the vehicle for the entire trip back to the police station. He had opened and closed every storage compartment within reach of his driving position. The ashtray only contained empty confectionery wrappers. The centre console between the two front seats was filled with an assortment of odds and ends that the owner had used at some point in time, or carried them with the prospect they may be needed sometime in the future. A small box of tissues was just the right size to fit into an indentation in the front dash on the passenger side. The rear seat had a booster seat secured on either side. A sundry of children's items were scattered all around. Small toys, clothing, a single shoe, and empty potato chip packets were amongst the discarded debris. Everything as it should be for a car with a young family to transport.

One item disturbed Ricky, though, and it dangled from the centre rear vision mirror. It constantly attracted Ricky's attention as his eyes flashed from the roadway to it. Elvis, dressed in a white sequinned jump suit, would bounce and jiggle with every bump and turn made by the four-wheel-drive.

Elvis was supported in mid-air by a length of string, just underneath the mirror. The string attached to the back of the plastic figure just below the neck.

Ricky couldn't help but wonder if this had been a source of inspiration for Reginald's method of suicide.

Ricky parked the vehicle. All Elvis could manage now was a slight sway. Ricky half expected to hear the groan of the string, just as the rope had done on the tree limb. However, all remained quiet.

Tombstone leaned across to the open passenger window of the police truck and called towards Ricky as he stretched out of the small four-wheel-drive. 'Jump in.'

Ricky walked over and stuck his head inside the police vehicle and replied, 'I was just going to get all his property and this car entered up.'

'Leave it until we get back,' said Tombstone in a tone that Ricky knew was pointless arguing with.

They should have knocked off over an hour ago, but Ricky knew Tombstone would want to attend the home of the deceased and deliver the death message to the man's wife. Ricky new better than to suggest the afternoon shift could do it. Tombstone would see the job through to the end, which included delivering the hardest message of all. It was police protocol to deliver all death messages face to face, and under no circumstances should it be done over the phone.

Ricky pulled himself up into the passenger seat of the police truck and remained silent for the three minutes it took to arrive at the deceased man's home. There was no need for conversation, as both officers were filled with dread of the task ahead.

Ricky and Tombstone could hear children's laughter as they stood outside the front door of the late Reginald Boyd's home. Ricky could not imagine how many of these messages Tombstone must have delivered over his career. He noticed, though, that Tombstone still had to prepare himself for the unpleasant task. He watched Tombstone take a noticeably deep breath while holding his eyes closed, or was it just an extra-long blink, Ricky could not decide. Upon opening his eyes, Tombstone gave a solid wrap to the timber door with his knuckles.

The laughter from inside stopped. Little feet were then heard running as a small voice yelled, 'Mummy, mummy. Someone's at the door.'

An attractive young woman opened the door. 'Oh,' was her initial, surprised reaction. It was quickly followed by a happy and smiling 'Hello.'

'Mrs. Boyd is it?' Tombstone asked cheerfully, not wanting to alarm the woman more than their presence had already done.

'Yes, that's right,' she replied a little reservedly, with no inkling of what was to come.

Tombstone introduced himself and Ricky, and then asked if they could come in. She happily obliged, albeit she was somewhat confused as to why the police would want to speak with her. She had never done anything wrong in her life.

'Can I get you gentlemen a cup of tea or coffee?' she asked as she ushered the two officers into the living room and invited them to take a seat.

Tombstone declined the offer. To assist with breaking the news, he could have done with something a little stronger to fortify his courage.

Two small boys joined their mother on the lounge. There naturally happy, youthful exuberance was now suppressed. The appearance of police can be intimidating for some adults, let alone a four and three-year old. The children's presence made Tombstone very uncomfortable.

'Is it possible to speak with you alone?' he suggested.

The wife hesitantly agreed. Her confusion was slowly turning to concern as she sent the two boys to play in a bedroom.

'Have I done something wrong?' she asked.

It was obvious she had no idea their presence was due to her husband. In some small way it contributed to the investigation into his death. It was a sign that she did not immediately fear the worst. If she had, then it could have indicated problems in the marriage or that deep down she was expecting this day to come.

Tombstone remained cheerful in his approach in order to glean as much information as he could before delivering the fatal news. 'No, nothing like that,' he replied. 'I just need to ask you some questions, that's all.'

'About what?' she asked directly.

Tombstone ignored the question. 'Firstly, do you have any relatives in town?' Tombstone was hoping that she or her husband had family close by. He would have them attend to comfort her in her grief to come.

'No. All our family is in Sydney. We've not long moved here for my husband's work.'

Tombstone recognised the woman and children from the photograph in the deceased's wallet, but still asked, 'Is your husband Reginald Arthur Boyd?'

'Yes that's right, but everyone calls him Reggie.' The woman's face appeared to light up as she mentioned his name.

'Is he home at the moment?' asked Tombstone pointedly.

'No. He's on afternoon shift at the fruit processing plant. He won't be home until midnight,' she replied, unaware of his fate.

Ricky looked around the living room that he found to be neat and tidy. He noticed some Elvis Presley memorabilia in a glass display cabinet.

Tombstone still had a long list of questions in his mind to ask. He wanted to know about her husband's general wellbeing, state of mind, marital problems, money problems, medication he may have been on, and a multitude of others. They would all be asked later. Tombstone now saw his opportunity to break the life changing news.

'I'm sorry to tell you, Mrs. Boyd…' Tombstone paused as he felt the hurt he was about to cause, 'But your husband won't be coming home tonight.'

'Oh no, has he injured himself at work?' she said, alarmed.

'Your husband never made it to work, Mrs. Boyd. Your husband died today.'

The widow was motionless. Her body frozen with the multitude of emotions that now coursed through her. Her piercing stare slowly moved onto Ricky as if seeking confirmation of what she was just told. It had to be wrong.

He shook his head slowly and held her gaze. 'I'm sorry, Mrs. Boyd.'

'How did it happen?' she asked without emotion after a moment's silence that felt like eternity.

Tombstone calmly told her the circumstances of her husband's suicide. When he finished, tears swelled in the woman's eyes. The flood quickly followed. Tombstone held her as her body began to slump onto the lounge. Tombstone did not utter another word for ten minutes. He just held on, trying to absorb as much of her pain as possible.

Ricky heard one of the children enter the room behind him. He quickly rose to his feet and approached the small boy. 'Hey tiger,' he said and held out a friendly hand towards the boy. 'Why don't you show me what you have been playing with?'

The child hesitated, then trustingly took hold of Ricky's hand and turned back towards the bedroom. He excitedly yelled out to his younger brother, 'Billy, the policeman wants to play with us.'

5PM

Bryan had all south-bound traffic stopped, fifty metres up the road from Lindsay's car. Rowdy had made the request in order to provide a safe work environment for him and the funeral contractors while they removed Lindsay's body from the car. To avoid anyone seeing the removal process, Rowdy had the fire personnel hold a tarp in a semicircle around the driver's side. Rowdy and the contractors could now work out of sight and without fear of being struck by passing traffic.

Lindsay's head was slumped forward, his chin rested on his chest. His skull was splayed open. Congealing blood and brain matter oozed forward and dripped from his forehead. With the driver's door wide open, Rowdy manoeuvred his arms behind Lindsay's back until he could cup a hand under each armpit. One contractor bent down and encircled his arms around Lindsay's legs until he could firmly clutch both hands together behind the knees.

On the count of three, both men heaved. Fortunately Lindsay was not a big man, which made the effort more manageable. They swung Lindsay's body out and up. The second contractor was standing with the gurney parallel to the car, giving the two lifters enough room to work. With Lindsay in mid-air, the contractor now pushed the trolley closer. The momentum of the swing landed Lindsay onto the gurney which was already lined with a tagged body bag.

Rowdy was relieved to see that the remainder of Lindsay's brain matter remained inside his shattered skull. It wobbled like jelly as Lindsay was straightened and tucked into the bag. The four firemen holding the tarp were all peering over its top edge while they removed the body. As if choreographed with military precision, they raised the tarp a little higher to cover their own eyes. Their initial morbid interest had now turned to revulsion as they reeled from the sight.

The contractors wheeled the gurney to the far edge of the breakdown lane to distance themselves from the highway so traffic could resume flowing. They were yet to do up the zipper so the firemen shuffled with the tarp and matched the contractor's movements.

Rowdy gave Bryan a wave to let the traffic go. He then turned his attention back to Lindsay. He patted him down as he would search an offender. He removed a wrist watch and wedding band, then pulled Lindsay's hips to one side to gain access to his rear trouser pocket and removed a wallet. The last item Rowdy removed was the mobile phone. All would be entered up on his return to Benstown Police Station and returned to family as soon as possible.

The funeral contractor zipped up the bag then pulled two straps across it, firmly securing it to the gurney. They didn't want Lindsay rolling out of bed in transit. The firemen lowered their tarp and began to fold it neatly along the existing crease marks.

Bryan returned from his traffic control duties and waited until the funeral contractors were out of ear shot. 'Once the body snatchers get their claws in they really don't want them getting away do they?' he said to Rowdy, in reference to the straps placed around the body.

With the body removed, the connection Rowdy felt was broken and he was now keen to leave the scene. 'That's it folks, parties over,' he said to the fireman as he removed his gloves. 'Thanks for all the help.'

The fire crew acknowledged Rowdy's appreciation and started to stow away their equipment. He turned to Bryan and Baz. 'I'll get you two to wait here for the tow truck. I'm off,' he said.

Bryan knew Rowdy was well past his knockoff time. He also knew how he would be feeling, in particular, that sense of ownership of a scene. In good humour, he could not help sharing one last insult with his colleague. 'That's right, give us the mop and bucket to clean up your mess,' he said with a serious tone.

Rowdy smiled at his friend and gave him an affectionate pat to one shoulder. 'Look at it this way, at least I can trust you with the mop and bucket.

A car horn sounded. The three officers looked around to see Mel about to pull out and enter the flow of traffic. She gave a wave through the windscreen that the officers returned. Rowdy made a mental note to submit a report to his commander about Mel's actions at the scene. He would request that she at least receive a Command Commendation in recognition for the assistance that she rendered.

Rowdy had only taken several steps towards his Highway Patrol car when the mobile phone he still held in his hand, with Lindsay's other possessions, stopped him in his tracks. On this occasion, the upbeat Mexican Hat Dance failed to brighten his spirits. He looked at the illuminated screen and read the name Mark. Over and over, Rowdy heard the voice in his head telling him not to answer the call.

'Hello,' Rowdy said as the phone pressed against his ear.

'Hi Dad,' answered Mark's voice.

Mark's flight had arrived several hours early. He had been trying to contact his parents to let them know. Rowdy immediately cursed his decision. He threw his head backwards and let out an audible sigh.

'Sorry, this is the police,' said Rowdy as his mind raced for words.

Before Rowdy could say another word, Mark immediately replied with concern. 'What's wrong? Where are my parents?'

'There currently unavailable at the moment.' Rowdy could not believe he used that stereotyped unanswered phone call response, but his mind fumbled to find the right words.

'Where are you?' he asked, deflecting the volley of questions from Mark.

The dread in Mark's voice travelled strongly across the digital signal. 'I'm waiting at Sydney Airport for my parents to pick me up. What's happened to them?' he demanded.

Rowdy knew he could not pass on the news of his father's death over the phone. From experience, Rowdy had learnt that there is no easy way or suitable time to inform someone of a loved one's death, but this certainly was not the time, or place.

'They've been in a car accident and…' he managed to say before being cut short by Mark's frantic voice.

'Are they okay?'

'They're okay,' lied Rowdy. 'But they have been taken to hospital.'

'How badly injured are they?' persisted Mark as he searched for answers.

Rowdy ignored the question. 'I'm going to have police meet you at the airport and convey you to your parents.'

Mark fired off another salvo of questions in quick succession. 'Where are they? What hospital?'

Rowdy again would not be drawn in to answer the questions directly. 'It will all be explained to you when the police pick you up.'

Rowdy kept on talking to take control of the conversation and to prevent Mark from asking any further questions. Any that he did ask, Rowdy continued to ignore. He told Mark where to meet the police and obtained his mobile phone number in case he could not retrieve it from Lindsay's phone.

The call was terminated and Rowdy made a bee line to his vehicle, not stopping to explain the phone conversation to Bryan and Baz. His only concern now was to convince the Duty Operations Inspector to have police run a taxi service for Mark. He was confident he would get his own way, but if he failed, he would drive to Sydney himself, on his own time if need be.

Ricky and Tombstone sat in the muster room of Chifley Police Station after having delivered the death message.

'It's hard to believe that someone could have no idea about how their spouse was truly feeling,' Ricky contemplated out loud, as he sat at a desk completing exhibit and miscellaneous property entries.

'Some people are good at hiding their emotions,' replied Tombstone, based on his own first hand knowledge of the subject.

Ricky still could not come to terms with how someone could live a double life. 'There has to be signs when you're living so close with someone,' he said.

'Do any of us slow down long enough to take notice of the signs?' Tombstone asked and gave Ricky more to contemplate. 'She said that he was always confident. Maybe there just weren't any indicators. As far as she was concerned, he left for work today just like any other day.'

'He must have felt completely overwhelmed to hang himself,' stated Ricky. He tried to think of something that would cause him to consider such a drastic act. He again came up empty on the thought.

'Don't rule out the possibility that all his problems could have been imagined,' Tombstone said to his young offsider. 'What you imagine to be true becomes your reality,' he added.

Ricky was surprised at Tombstone's response. 'Where did you learn that? Psych 101?'

Tombstone's face was lined with experience. He added to its creases as his face broadened into a grin. It was directed more at himself than at Ricky. His young offsider still thought learning was something that came from books. Tombstone had a better teacher.

'No, I learnt that after dealing with people and all their problems over the last twenty five years.'

Ricky paused from his bookwork and studied Tombstone's craggy face. He wondered what he had seen in those twenty five years. One thing he knew for sure, he would never hear about it from this mostly private man. It was a rare occasion to hear Tombstone recount old war stories from the job. Ricky's admiration and respect for the veteran officer continued to grow with each shift working with him.

Ricky averted his eyes back to his work as Tombstone, who was sitting at a desk opposite, lifted his own head. His deep brown eyes narrowed as he appraised Ricky and was satisfied that the young officer had potential. Not only did he ask annoying questions, he was always thinking about his work.

Ricky slapped closed the exhibit book. 'Done,' he exclaimed and glanced at his wrist watch to check if he could still make it to his squash competition. 'Looks like I forfeited the squash game,' he added with regret.

Tombstone could not help himself. He had to make the most of the opportunity that Ricky just presented. 'Not to worry,' he said from a stony face without looking up from his work. 'I hear you're not that good, so you probably would have lost anyway.'

Ricky absorbed the good natured insult. The reality was, the comment was fairly accurate. He tossed the dead man's jewellery and belongings into a bag and labelled it with the reference number. The suicide note, that he had just finished entering into the Exhibit Book, was also bagged and tagged.

'Have you got much left to do?' he asked Tombstone as a way of offering to help.

'No. I've finished the P79A so it can get to the Coroner in the morning. The rest can wait for another day.'

The afternoon shift Station Officer stuck his head around the door of the muster room. 'Call for you Tombstone,' he said.

Tombstone was already two hours overdue to knock off. 'Tell them I've finished work for the day.'

'She said she spoke with you not long ago about that dead guy's wife,' added the Station Officer to emphasise the importance.

'Alright, put her through to 601,' replied Tombstone, leaning across the desk to check the telephone extension number.

Prior to leaving the home of the deceased's wife, Tombstone had telephoned one of her friends who lived nearby. Tombstone and Ricky had stayed at the house until she arrived. He had no idea why she would be calling now.

The telephone beside Tombstone came to life. He picked up the receiver on the first ring. After greeting the lady, he remained silent while she spoke. She was asking for help on how to deal with her good friend's loss.

'I'm sorry but I didn't know who else to call. I've never had to help anyone grieving like this before,' her voice quaked over the telephone line.

'I'm no expert on grief counselling,' Tombstone started to say. In actual fact, he was probably more qualified to give advice than any counsellor with a university degree. He continued hesitantly, unsure what he could offer the woman. 'All you can do is support her and the kids.'

'But how do I do that? I don't want to say the wrong thing.'

'Be a very good listener,' replied Tombstone. 'Talk about her loss when you think the time is right. It will probably be more uncomfortable for you to do that than it will be for her.' Tombstone shared his experience. 'Hold her if she needs holding, or just sit with her in silence if that's what she is after. Just being around can help. It lets her know that people care about her and are not avoiding her. She may feel lost and find it hard to do everyday mundane things so help out with those two kids or do the housework and shopping for her.'

'You make it sound so easy,' said the woman's voice as it echoed through the phone.

Tombstone tried to lighten the mood and said with a light laugh, 'It's always easy when you're on this side of the phone.'

The woman's voice seemed to brighten. 'Thank you for your advice,' she said warmly from the heart.

'Anytime,' replied Tombstone.

The woman now managed a laugh of her own and said, 'I'll get a big pot of soup on tonight to put in her freezer.'

'Now you're getting the hang of it,' said Tombstone and passed on his goodbyes.

Ricky had been listening to the one sided conversation. 'Is everything alright.'

Tombstone returned the telephone handpiece to its cradle. 'It will be….in time.'

Dick and Ben had gone about the rest of their work with little need for communication between them. They had finished recording the scene at the fiery fatal, and Ben was loading some of his equipment back into his forensic van.

Inspector Rob Cooley had left, which meant Dick was back in charge of the scene as the ranking officer. The Duty Officer was on his way to Brookstone Police Station to send off a sit-rep of the incident to the Regional Commander's Office in Kingstown. The situation report would give the Regional Commander and his Staff Officer a brief but concise overview of the scene and the actions taken by police. There would, no doubt, be media interest in the collision and the sit-rep would more than likely be passed onto the Police Media Liaison Officer to inform all media outlets of the facts. Given its horrific nature, Dick was surprised that no media had arrived at the scene. He could not imagine what else may have happened in the area to take precedence over this tragedy.

He was not disappointed, it was one less complication to deal with. It must be his lucky day after all, he thought to himself.

Standing next to the burnt-out car, Dick took a moment and surveyed the scene. For the first time he could view the scene in its entirety now that his peripheral vision had well and truly returned. The surrounding land had been scorched black. He cast his eyes down the gentle grade of the Great North Highway towards the jack-knifed semi. The remaining police and fire personnel had little to do until Dick and Ben completed their work, and they still just looked on in silence. No emotions flooded him as he took in the carnage of the wreckage and the gore of its victim. Intermittently, the smell of charred flesh was carried to his nostrils on the light breeze. All Dick could think was how peaceful everything now seemed.

Dick prolonged his gaze over the destruction of man and machine. This carnage was Dick's sense of normality and was the only place he felt in control. This normality came at a price, though, and Dick was blinded to the heavy toll it was extracting from him.

His moment of serenity was disturbed by the rush of air, followed by a grinding squeal as the driver of a heavy lift tow truck applied his air brakes. The large rigid finally came to a jolting rest with a final burst of air that left its tow hitch mounted on the back swinging. Dick casually turned and walked towards it.

The driver of the tow truck jumped down from his high cabin. The short, tight shorts that he wore threatened to expose his manhood. His padded build amply filled the faded blue singlet, worn like a uniform for many truck drivers. His landing was cushioned by the ten millimetres of rubber that were the soles of his thongs, or 'work boots' as some may call them in the transport industry. With a quick hitch up of his shorts under his impressive beer gut, he still failed to cover the vertical cleft that divided his gluteus maximus.

'How are ya mate?' the cheery truck driver greeted Dick from several metres away. The man's stride was restricted by a reserve of fat that devoured his knees. His short stature waddled more than walked. 'What have ya got for me?'

Dick turned his upper body as he walked towards the truck driver and pointed behind at the jack-knifed truck.

'That burnt out shell down there is all yours.'

'She good to go?' asked the tow truck driver, referring to the truck in the feminine gender.

He couldn't help but pick up on the female reference. He pointed towards the tarp that once again partly covered the burnt out car containing the decapitated driver and replied, 'Yes, she is. But watch her, she could be a femme fatale given the result of this bloke's attraction to her.'

A blank look appeared on the tow truck driver's face as he tried to decipher the comment, but to no avail. 'So, I can hitch her up?' he asked, to confirm whether he could take the semi-trailer.

'Yes, you can,' replied Dick, restraining himself from making any further comment about the truck's gender. 'There are some coppers down there with...' Dick stopped himself from saying 'her' and instead finished with... 'it.'

'Thanks mate,' said the tow truck driver and turned on his rubber heels and flip flopped his way back to his truck.

Just as the heavy lift tow truck pulled away; it was replaced with a smaller one. It had arrived to take the burnt out car to the police holding yard for mechanical examination. Dick passed on the news to the truck driver that he would have to wait until they removed the body.

Dick approached Ben as he was lifting the tarp covering the half slice of head and other facial bits and pieces. The two officers stood side by side looking down at the one eyed monster that stared back at them.

'I'll toss you for it,' Dick said without looking at Ben.

'Tell you what,' replied Ben casually. 'Hold the bag while I lift it up.'

He smiled briefly as he noticed Ben called the man's face it. 'Sounds good to me.'

Dick removed one of several plastic bags he had stuffed into his thigh pocket. Both officers snapped on a pair of latex gloves and crouched down beside the face. He spread the bag open as far as it would stretch and held it towards Ben.

Without hesitation, Ben took hold of the man's ebony hair and peeled the scalp towards him. The soggy, meaty tissue underneath made a slurping sound as its suction with the road was broken. Ben peeled the face clear of the roadway, and then flipped it like a pancake to rest on one hand. His fingers were fully splayed to create a larger surface area. The shredded edges of the face still drooped over his hand. Ben studied the underside and flicked off the odd small piece of road aggregate that stuck to its flesh. Ben was fascinated at what he saw. '

You can still see the optic nerve running to the back of the eye,' he pointed out and moved his hand closer for Dick to see.

'That's good Ben… just put it in the bag.'

Ben delicately slid the face inside the bag that Dick immediately sealed. He then placed the bag onto the road and removed another from his pocket. The pair moved onto the cheek and jaw fragment. Ben's morbid fascination continued as he scrutinised each of the next four items that they gathered.

With the last and smallest of the human flesh portions now bagged, the two officers had one last task to perform. As if on cue, an unmarked white van pulled up behind Ben's forensic van. The only occupant of the van was the driver.

'There like circling vultures,' Dick said in reference towards the funeral contractor. 'They only land when it's safe to pick at the carcass.'

5.30PM

Ricky swung the door of his locker closed after hanging up his appointment belt and returning his police cap to the shelf inside. Without needing to change out of his police uniform for the short trip home, Ricky grabbed his sports bag and headed for the door of the change room.

Before he could clear the door, his progress was cut short by the appearance of the Station Sergeant, whose generous stature and physique filled the doorway.

'I didn't know you were still here, sarge?' said Ricky.

The Station Sergeant's rumbling voice matched his appearance, big and rough. 'I was just about to say the same about you.'

'Not for much longer,' replied Ricky. 'I'm heading off now.'

The big Station Sergeant made no effort to clear a path for the young officer. 'You've had a big day,' he stated.

'Yeah, Tombstone and I managed to fill in our time,' said Ricky and took a small step towards the doorway, thinking the Station Sergeant would stand aside. He did not.

'I just wanted to check in with you,' the big sergeant said and crossed his arms on his chest and leaned against the door jamb to indicate he was not going anywhere. 'See how you're feeling.'

Ricky could see he wasn't going anywhere just yet. He placed his sports bag onto the table in the middle of the small room.

'Feeling?' Ricky asked with surprise. 'I'm feeling fine. A bit pissed off I missed my squash game though,' he finished with a chuckle.

The Station Sergeant's normally rough tone now softened and he said with obvious concern in his voice, 'Those two deadens you had today can often fill you with many conflicting feelings.'

'Really Sarge, I'm fine,' said Ricky reassuringly. 'It was my first cot death and Tombstone taught me a lot today.'

'He said you did well today,' commented the Station Sergeant, passing on the compliment that he knew Tombstone would never do.

Ricky smiled as the compliment filled him with pride. 'Thanks, that's good to hear.'

'I just wanted to remind you that it's normal to have a mixture of emotions after experiencing what you did today.'

The old Station Sergeant had seen many dedicated police officers crumble under the strain of emotional stress. He knew that police of all generations, as well as other emergency personnel, liked to portray themselves as tough. Too professional to let their work affect them. The experienced officer knew the truth, though. He knew they felt that families and friends in other professions were unable to completely understand their experiences. It was these shared experiences that formed the strong bond between police. Even though they may not call themselves friends, they share a sturdy and faithful connection simply because of the job they do.

'Just remember,' the Station Sergeant continued in a soft tone never heard by the general public. 'I'm here to talk about anything if you need to.'

The Station Sergeant did not know it, but what he was actually doing was referred to by mental health professionals as *defusing*. It is the initial stage of the debriefing process after being exposed to a critical incident. It should always be done the day of the incident and before the person exposed has had a chance to sleep. The old Sergeant had unknowingly performed this task better than if he had recited it out of a manual.

Unlike his Station Sergeant, Ricky started to feel a bit embarrassed and uncomfortable with the conversation. He grabbed his sports bag and repeated himself, 'Really sarge, I'm fine.'

This time, when Ricky moved forward, the Station Sergeant lumbered sideways and back from the doorway, making just enough room for Ricky to pass.

The Station Sergeant waited until Ricky had taken several steps past when he said, 'Just one more thing, Ricky.'

Ricky stopped and turned with an enquiring look. The Station Sergeant answered his look with the return of the usual coarseness in his voice. 'You will be required to attend a debrief.'

The purpose of a debrief is to allow the person, or even a group of people to talk about a specific incident within seventy-two hours of its occurrence. It is carried out without judgement or criticism as the emphasis is always about keeping people safe. It helps them to quickly return to a more normal level of functioning, albeit, at a new level of normal.

Ricky physically slumped at the prospect of attending a process he just did not believe in. 'Do I have to?' he queried. 'I've been to worse and never had a debrief before.'

'Yes,' said the Station Sergeant with added harshness.

'But….' Ricky started to protest but was cut short.

'Attendance is mandatory,' insisted the Station Sergeant in a no-nonsense tone, and then paused before adding, 'On the other hand, participation is not.'

Ricky resigned himself to the fact he would be attending. 'Will Tombstone be there?' he asked.

'No, Tombstone and I will be meeting later with Dr. Toohey for his debrief.'

Ricky thought nothing more of this last comment as he left for home. What he did not know was that Tombstone was a so-called functioning alcoholic who had turned to the bottle to numb the pain he felt from so many years working on the front line. His nerves were shattered beyond repair.

Uncharacteristically, for the second time within a short passage of time, Dick's temper flared immediately. 'You're kidding me,' he said with astonishment, as the funeral contractor informed him of the news. 'You're it.'

The funeral contractor shrugged his shoulders. 'It's all part of the boss's new cost cutting measures. Only one staff member per callout.'

Dick turned his head to the sky in disbelief and swivelled away from the man standing in front of him. When facing in the opposite direction, he stopped and lowered his head. His eyes fell upon the decapitated, charcoaled human form still sitting behind the steering wheel of the car. His hopes of not being involved in the body's removal crumbled.

The funeral contractor had his hands deep into his trouser pockets when Dick turned back to face him. The man's head was bowed to the ground as he took great interest in the roadway that he tortured under the ball of one foot. From the contractor's obviously embarrassed stance, Dick knew there was more bad news to come.

'So how are you going to get your customer out of his car?' demanded Dick in an uncontrolled harsh tone, knowing full well what the answer would be.

The uncomfortable funeral contractor took a step back. He feared his answer may incite the officer to lash out at him. 'Well…' he paused while he chose his words carefully. 'The thing is…' His words only stumbled out. No matter how he phrased his reply, the result was going to be the same. 'Because our boss has made this decision to only send one man per callout, our union has reacted by taking industrial action.'

Even though the contractor looked everywhere except at Dick, he could still feel Dick's glare burning a hole into his forehead.

'And what industrial action would that be?' asked Dick now with a consciously controlled calmness that did not reflect the multitude of expletives that flowed through his mind.

The funeral contractor noticeably squirmed as he tried to shift the blame. 'Our union has told us to refuse to lift anything heavy.'

'And what does your union class as… heavy?' he asked, calling on all his will power to remain calm.

The funeral contractor now studied the road as if looking for a hole to crawl into. He replied meekly. 'Bodies.'

It was solely the amusement factor that now kept Dick talking. In some way it managed to calm him internally. 'So you're telling me that you're in the business of collecting bodies but you can't collect them.'

'I can still collect the body,' the contractor replied quickly, wrongly believing Dick was confused. He now met Dick's hostile gaze. 'I just can't physically pick it up. Our union…'

Dick cut the man off. 'I know, your union said so. Who is going to pick up the slack, so to speak?' He asked and assumed an aggressive stance to match his facial expression by placing his clenched fists onto his hips.

The funeral contractor now had real fear on his face and stuttered, 'Our… our… our union said, in the…the meantime, get the police to lift the bodies.'

Although Dick was never much of a union man, it never ceased to amaze him how strong and militant other occupations' unions could be in order to achieve the best outcome for their rank and file members. His own Police Associations idea of forcing the government's hand was to threaten them that police would *Work to Rules*. This was a reference to the Police Rules and Instructions book which set out in black and white how police should do their job. He could think of nothing more absurd.

His union would basically say to the government that if they did not give the police what they wanted, then they would stuff the whole system up by performing their duties in accordance with the rule book.

Dick took a quick step towards the funeral contractor. At the same time he raised a fist forward from its resting place on his hip. On seeing the movement, the contractor's eyes widened as large as dinner plates. He started to turn away to avoid the blow that he felt was surely coming. He moved too slowly though. His movement was barely past the thought stage when Dick landed a heavy but open hand onto the man's shoulder.

'Happy to help your cause out,' said Dick in a cheery voice, and a transformed face to match.

The funeral contractor slumped with relief. He lowered his head again, but this time it was not to avoid Dick's eyes. He had to double check there was no damp stain spreading across the front of his trousers.

'Leave it to us,' Dick continued, managing to turn his hostile mood around with the acceptance of the task. He patted the contractor's shoulder playfully. 'You just bring your trolley over, Ben and I will do the heavy lifting for you.'

Ford was now within earshot, having finished packing his crime scene equipment away. He carried the bags of body parts as casually as he would the grocery shopping.

'What will Ben do?' he asked as he moved closer.

Dick informed Ben of the situation with the funeral contractor.

'I couldn't think of anything I'd rather do at the moment,' said Ben, apparently happy to get the charred body out of the car. He then extended his hand holding the plastic bags towards the contractor. 'These are for you.'

The funeral contractor took the bags and examined, with a look of disgust, the face in side profile. Its moist flesh had covered most of the bag inside with a slimy coating, which had already started to turn green.

'Some days I really wonder why I do this job,' remarked the funeral contractor as he headed off towards his van.

Dick and Ben could only look at each other and shake their heads in bewilderment at the hard-done-by funeral contractor.

Within ten minutes, the fire personnel had cut the roof off the burnt-out car. The driver's door also lay discarded on the roadway to give Dick better access to the body.

'How do you want to do this?' Dick asked Ben.

Both officers were now dressed in a pair of disposable overalls and stood side by side at the car looking at the headless body.

'I've always been a leg man myself,' Ben replied as he studied the charred, blackened remains. 'You can take the shoulders.'

Each man manoeuvred themselves into position and braced to lift the dead weight. Dick shuffled his feet a little wider to steady himself against the impending lift. Ben gave a count to three, then both men lifted in unison. The force they exerted was much more than required and the surprisingly light weight of the body was reflected on their faces. Dick was hoping to raise the stiffened body just clear of the steel seat frame and his astonishment was vocalised with a groan when he nearly tossed the body into the air.

'Well I guess he is only half the man he used to be,' joked Ben.

Ben was right. With clothing, flesh and much of his muscle tissue burnt, the man's weight was greatly reduced. The two officers repositioned themselves. Dick stood with his gloved hands under what was left of the man's armpits. From his position, Dick was looking straight down at the severed neck. Thankfully the fire had cauterised the wound into a crusty mess that resembled melted plastic.

They started to move the rigid body from the vehicle, but progress was soon halted when the uncooperative corpse refused to let go of the steering wheel. The hands were nearly reduced to bone but still had enough sinew to hold them firmly clutching the steering wheel. They returned the modern day headless horseman to his seat. Ben delicately forced each finger straight. The remaining flesh was bubbled like pork crackling and just as crispy. The sound was like ribs being torn apart to separate them. Ben expected the fingers to snap off, but none did.

The pair lifted a third time and cleared the body from the car. They then stopped as they looked perplexingly at the waiting trolley, then back at the body. The man was mummified in his driving posture. His seared arms still outstretched, having only sagged slightly when the hands left the steering wheel. The man's entire body was roasted and had a hard rough texture to it. What Ben held in his cupped hands was shrivelled up thighs which stuck out at right angles from the torso. The lower legs bent at the knees and hung, still reaching for the accelerator and brake.

The corpse reminded Dick of figures he had seen in books of victims unearthed in Pompeii. Men, women, and dogs preserved how they lay as ash and poisonous gases consumed them.

'We'll just have to put him on as he is,' said Dick.

Ben gave a moment's thought then said, 'If you can hold him, I'll see if his legs will go down a bit.'

Dick leant his body backwards as he braced against the force Ben exerted when he pushed down on the dead man's knees. The legs barely moved. Ben applied more downward pressure and could now hear the crackle of burnt tissue as it tore and split at the hips. The charred flesh left covering the man's stomach suddenly ripped open like a ripe watermelon being cut. The body had been so deeply burnt that the stomach, intestines, and other internal organs were just below the surface of the scorched tissue. The intense heat had penetrated into the body and cooked the organs to the point that their tough fibrous tissue had been compromised.

A flood of digestive juices, food in various stages of digestion, and a thick brown food paste burst out through the tear. The human soup came with such a rush that Ben, who was standing directly in front of the body and partly between the legs, couldn't move out of the way quickly enough. He jumped backwards, leaving Dick holding the corpse.

Before Ben knew what was happening, his disposable overalls, where they bloused over his footwear, were drenched in the putrid mix. His polished black boots covered in a slime of bodily fluids. Ben was stunned as he looked down at his soiled clothing. All he could do was stand there with arms outstretched from his side while his face screwed up, making him look like the most forlorn figure anyone could see.

Dick continued to hold the lightweight corpse in front of him then propped it against an outstretched thigh. He felt for his colleague, but inwardly thanked whatever superior being was listening that it wasn't him standing there covered in offal. Dick finally broke the silence when he said to Ben, 'Well that beats being covered in fleas.'

Rowdy stretched back from his office desk in his chair. The furnishings of the Highway Patrol Office in Benstown Police Station could only be described as eclectic. No two desks and chairs matched. The only thing all the office furniture had in common was it looked tired and worn. Filing cabinets looked like they had just come straight from the dump, with pre-loved dents and scratches.

The drawers had long ago worn out their rollers and required a hard fought battle to wrestle them open. Some had fought their last battle and just remained open, never to close again. In the end it was easier to use whatever desk and floor space available to file documents, just to avoid the conflict of fighting with the cabinet.

To persist in their use would only result in further dents as force born from frustration was used to encourage them to open or close.

As Rowdy leaned back looking at the stained yellow ceiling that dated back to an era when smoking was an acceptable pastime indoors, he rubbed the open palm of both hands up and down his tired face, massaging his weary eyes. It had been a long day.

He was pleased that prior to leaving the scene of Lindsay's collision, he had convinced the Duty Operations Inspector to have police in Sydney attend the airport.

They would inform Mark of his father's death and then start the relay to have him escorted to his mother.

Rowdy glanced at the askew wall clock. Ten minutes to six. He let out a sigh and straightened in his chair to return his focus to the computer screen, whose cursor blinked impatiently for its next command. He was due at his children's school play in ten minutes. He was not going to make it. With at least another twenty minutes work to tidy up his day, he then had to drive the twenty minutes down to Bowen and the children's school. His mind started to work out the apology speech to Emma and the kids.

Rowdy was tearing the last of the tickets from his infringement book when he heard the rear door of the police station creak open. It was quickly followed by the boisterous conversation, mixed with laughter, of Bryan and Baz. The pair entered the office as Rowdy leaned across and slipped his tickets into a mailing tray that sat atop one of the damaged filing cabinets.

'I thought you would have been gone by now,' Bryan said, surprised to see Rowdy still at his desk. 'Milking the overtime I see.'

Rowdy had not even considered claiming overtime. He gave it a quick thought and then disregarded it. For one thing, he could not be bothered typing out the claim form and extending his day further. Secondly, he did not want to explain why he stayed longer at the scene than he had to without getting a Duty Officer to recommend and approve the overtime.

'You know me Bryan,' replied Rowdy. 'Do it for the love of the job.'

'Love doesn't pay the bills though,' Baz scoffed.

Rowdy started to enter Lindsay's property into the Miscellaneous Property Book. 'Did the scene get cleaned up alright?' he asked Bryan.

Bryan was taking a seat in a swivel chair whose foam padding had long lost its comfortable qualities. He leant back and placed his feet against the edge of a desk. Baz chose the more agreeable corner of a desktop to plant his behind.

'Yeah,' answered Bryan as he squirmed to get comfortable. An unlit cigarette danced between his lips. 'The tow truck arrived only a minute after you left.'

Rowdy paused from the entry he was making in the property book and scribbled a note into his diary. He added to his 'to do' list the completion of a statement about Lindsay's accident that would be requested by the Crash Investigation Unit.

Bryan walked over to Rowdy and placed a single sheet of paper next to him. 'While you've got your pen out, fill in the seatbelt enforcement return with your figures. I'll fax it to the Region Office before I knock off tonight,' he said.

Rowdy quickly marked the numerous boxes asking for a breakdown of what infringements he had issued for the shift. The form also requested the number of charges laid during the shift and the number of breath tests performed.

'All this information about pro-active road safety, but they don't want to know how many people I killed this shift,' said Rowdy, even though he knew the Region Office had already been informed of the days fatalities by the numerous sit-reps that had been sent.

'I'll put that in the property room for you Rowdy,' Baz said, offering to help when he saw him securing Lindsay's personal items into an envelope and referencing the outside. 'It's time for you to go home.'

'That's the second best idea you've had today Baz,' replied Rowdy, and rose stiffly from his chair. He couldn't help wonder how the Safe-T-Cam data was going as he made his way out of the room.

6.00PM

The traffic on the Great North Highway was sparse as Dick continued his drive north, back to Brookstone. The afternoon peak-hour was over and the bank-up of traffic delayed by the accident scene had well and truly cleared. Dick had left the scene as Ben was having his boots hosed off by the fire brigade. Fortunately, the disposable overalls he was wearing at the time protected his uniform from the soaking of gastric juices that had spilled from the dead man's body.

He was not long into his journey before the intrusive thoughts that had plagued him all day, returned. He tried hard to focus on the roadway ahead but his mind controlled what his eyes saw and they focused on a very different image. Nightmares now invaded his waking hours.

Dick saw himself running. He could even feel the sensation of physical exertion as sweat began to bead down his temples over the pulsing skin caused by his increased heart rate once again. His breathing became louder as his lungs heaved to take in more oxygen to feed the starving muscles that his mind said were burning. Dick continued running, fearful of what pursued him. He glanced over one shoulder, without breaking stride, at the figure gaining on him. His arms pumped faster in a bid to generate more speed into his legs, but no matter how hard he tried, he could not outrun his pursuer.

In contrast to Dick's frantic toil, the rag doll that followed him covered the ground effortlessly. The rag doll was in human proportions and equalled Dick in size. Dick glanced once more over his shoulder. Even closer now, the rag doll partially transformed its appearance.

Dick's fear transformed along with it to sheer terror and he renewed his efforts to escape.

The inanimate head of the doll was now replaced with a human head. Exaggerated cross-stitch marks secured the head onto the wadded fabric body. The head let out a spine tingling cry as it came within arm's reach of Dick. Its padded arms rose out in front of its body. Human hands secured by the same cross-stitch pattern as on the neck clutched towards him. The harmless child's toy had turned into a monster of Frankenstein proportions. Another chilling shriek seemed to originate just millimetres away from his ear. The sound in his head was deafening.

Dick returned to reality with the suddenness of a falling dream just before landing. He panted for breath as the stretch of roadway before him came back into focus. A car travelling towards him suddenly materialised. His awareness had been so poor; he failed to see the car approaching from half a kilometre away that the sight distance on this span of road allowed. To Dick, it was as if the car had just driven through a time-warp and been placed on the road fifty metres away.

The oncoming car wandered within its lane slightly, towards the centre dividing line. Dick picked up on the movement but perceived it as an exaggerated swerve to the centre of the road. Dick instantly calculated the continued trajectory of the car would place it in the centre of his own vehicle. With both vehicles doing one-hundred kilometres an hour, all he saw was a collision of fatal proportions.

He reefed the steering wheel to the left. The police vehicle swerved violently, causing the tyres to howl in protest as they flexed and distorted, barely maintaining their grip on the roadway. Everything not secured inside the vehicle was tossed to one side as the centrifugal force tried to carry the vehicle and its contents in the opposite direction to which Dick steered.

The approaching car never crossed the centre line. Its wheels never even came close to touching the painted dividing marker and the imminent head-on collision that Dick anticipated passed without fruition. The other car continued on its journey, leaving its driver wondering why the police vehicle had swerved like it did. Its driver constantly checked his rear vision mirror after the two vehicles had passed. He was expecting to see the police vehicle thrown into a U-turn and come accelerating after him for some offence he was unaware of. Once in the breakdown lane and travelling straight again, the driver only saw brake lights illuminate on the rear of the police vehicle until it came to a jerking stop.

Dick gripped the steering wheel tensely, long after stopping. His head was pushed back into the padded seat as he sat with his eyes closed tightly. The sights and sounds of his imagined head-on collision would not leave him. He sat for the next five minutes, fighting for composure over the nervous wreck he was becoming.

This was the start of his hypersensitivity to sights and sounds which would progressively worsen over time. His everyday life would only continue to become more abnormal, but he still managed to convince himself that everything was alright. The fact that he felt normal when he was picking up body parts did not strike him as at all bizarre.

Rowdy walked out of the gun-safe room after unloading and securing his firearm. He headed in the direction of the change room and quickened his pace after checking the time on his wrist watch. He passed through the empty muster room, the main workstation area for the General Duty police. A narrow workstation bench ran the full length of a side wall. Three computer terminals were evenly spaced along its length. The rest of the bench area was decorated with a clutter of paper, folders, manuals, and useless junk that had not been used in six months. Everyone who used the area obviously worked on the theory that someone else was responsible for keeping it tidy.

In the centre of the opposite wall was an impressive marble fireplace with a timber mantle. The days when split timber would crackle in the hearth to provide winter warmth to the living room of the old residence that it once was, were long gone.

Cedar architraves, thirty centimetres wide, moulded their way around doorways and skirted the floor, only to be met by worn, soiled carpet. If anyone took the time to look up, they would see the craftsmanship of true tradesman continued on the high ceiling. Its decorative cedar panelling was a joinery masterpiece that sat atop the room as its crowning glory. The quality of the room was lost amongst the facsimile and photocopy machine. The metal cupboards and filing cabinets that filled any vacant space gave the room an industrial feel and it was treated as such.

The sight of a tastefully decorated, warm cosy room was lost to history. It was probably a sight that the younger police stationed there couldn't even imagine.

Rowdy had been told by the Duty Operations Inspector that the arrangements to pick Lynda Crisp's son, Mark, up at the airport had been made. He still felt uneasy – it was not that he failed to trust other people to organise things, he just had more faith in himself and less in others.

Before he made it through the muster room, he found himself seated behind one of the computer monitors, pushing aside a mountain of rubbish to find a buried telephone. He had to make the call to check the arrangements for Mark's transport were actually going ahead. If he did not, he knew that doubt would plague him all night.

Rowdy punched in the internal eaglenet number for the radio operations room in Kingstown. Before he heard the first ring tone he quickly pressed the receiver toggle to disconnect the call and held his finger on it while he considered his options. If he spoke with the DOI again, it would be easy for him to give lip service to the arrangements without actually checking. Rowdy needed independent confirmation to quell his distrust.

He flipped open a flap on a breast pocket and removed his notebook. He turned to the last page of writing and dialled the mobile phone number he had recorded. Mark answered. He was sitting in the back of a police sedan on the freeway heading north out of the city. He had been told of his father's death.

Relieved and satisfied, Rowdy replaced the telephone handpiece into its cradle. He inwardly told himself not to doubt others and to have confidence in their abilities, however, he knew he would do exactly the same again.

Within a minute of making the phone call to Mark, Rowdy was changed into his civilian clothes. He turned the key in his locker and noisily jiggled the handle to check it was locked. He bent down and picked up the old sports bag that was between his feet. In the same motion of straightening, he turned to his right to exit the change room. He stopped short as the officer working station duty on the afternoon shift entered.

'Hoping I'd find you here, Rowdy,' said the Station Officer.

Rowdy made an obvious point to check his wrist watch. 'What's up Mike?' he asked, hoping not to be asked to do anything else. He should have knocked off two and a half hours ago.

'I just got a call from the Duty Officer up at Brookstone. He wanted me to let you know that he will be organising a debrief for those deadens you attended today,' replied the officer.

Rowdy was slightly taken back by the message. It was totally unexpected. 'I've only ever had one debrief in my entire career. What makes the department so caring now?'

'Just passing on the message, Rowdy,' said Mike, at a loss to answer the question, and shrugging his shoulders.

Rowdy considered the information after getting over his initial surprise. While he was not against attending a debrief, he was slightly annoyed it would take time out of his already busy days.

'Did they say when it is?' Rowdy now asked.

Mike shook his head. 'They have to make the arrangements.'

'Thanks Mike. I'm back on tomorrow. I'll chase it up then,' Rowdy said as he walked past the officer and headed for the door.

Dick managed to make it safely back to Brookstone Police Station. After the scare he received from seeing himself involved in a head on collision, the remainder of the drive was completed wide eyed and with intense concentration. Just as he slumped into a chair behind his desk, Garry Harker entered the office and released his booming voice, 'I thought I saw you walk past my office door, Dick.'

Harker paced the carpet in front of Dick's desk. The office was not large but Dick was confident that the active detective sergeant would travel a kilometre during their conversation. Harker was a man who could not stand still. He was the epitome of perpetual motion, if harnessed, could solve the world's energy crisis. His hyperactivity may have had something to do with the cup of strong black coffee he held in his left hand. Even in those rare moments he did not have the mug in his hand, his fingers would still be curled around an imaginary handle.

Detective Sergeant Harker was not often referred to as a handsome man. It was joked around the station that the cartoonist for the animated feature film 'Shrek' just had to paint Garry's face green and the sketch of the ogre character was complete. Perhaps it was his less obvious qualities that people found attractive, after all, he was onto his third wife.

Garry did not bother to enquire why Dick was still at work. He just saw an opportunity. 'Dick, I need you to do a mouth swab on a bloke,' he bellowed, shooting balls of spittle from his mouth.

Dick rarely said no but today he was determined to make an exception. 'I knocked off at four-thirty, sarge. I shouldn't be here.'

'I'll approve the overtime,' persisted the detective.

'All the other police here have done the same mouth swab course that I've done,' Dick explained, hoping the detective would change his mind. 'Preventing overtime was the whole idea of training everyone to do the forensic procedure.'

Harker had not stopped pacing the whole time and now added his free hand to animate his conversation. 'It's for a murder investigation,' he added to reinforce the importance of the matter. 'I need someone who's not going to stuff it up. The only person capable of that is you.'

Dick looked puzzled. 'I didn't know we had a murder recently.'

'The request came from detectives at Coffs Harbour where the murder happened. The suspect lives here in Brookstone though,' Garry explained, and then had to wipe the back of his hand across the corners of his mouth to remove the foam that was building up as he spoke.

Dick desperately wanted to say no. 'Righto,' he said reluctantly. 'What time is this going to happen?'

Garry managed to look at his wrist watch without spilling a drop of coffee. The hand was nearing six-thirty. 'He should be coming through the door any minute now.'

Dick rose from his chair and reached into his pocket for a handkerchief to wipe a sniffling nose. 'I'd better get prepared then.'

Harker left the room as quickly as he arrived. His voice remained in the room, as he boomed from the corridor, 'I owe you one, Dick.'

Dick raised the hanky to his face. He caught a glimpse of a stain on the white linen, just before he covered his nose. Dick pulled the soiled fabric away from his face to focus on it better. Comprehension then struck him as he remembered wiping blood from his hands at the accident scene. With nowhere to discard the hanky at the time, Dick had placed it back into his pocket. He had not given it another thought since. Dick now screwed up his face and let the hanky dangle between the tips of his thumb and index fingers. He quickly discarded it into the rubbish bin and headed straight to the bathroom to scrub and disinfect his hands once more.

6.30PM

Rowdy was hesitant to enter. He felt himself hold his breath as he crossed the threshold into the packed multi-purpose centre at his children's school. When confronted with the mass of humanity inside, he audibly and involuntarily gasped. He had recently started to consciously avoid crowds. He was becoming increasingly agitated when surrounded by people. Even small social gatherings with family and friends were becoming harder to attend as he felt awkward and out of place.

He scanned the room, looking for his wife. If it was his choice, he would sit at the back of the auditorium where he could keep an eye on everyone else. An added bonus would be to sit near the exit door. It was not to be, however.

His wife Emma had been watching the entrance with increasing frustration.

Her husband was already half an hour late and their children were just about to take to the stage for the first time. A hand raised above the crowd, right in the centre of the room. Rowdy hoped it was an excited mother waving to one of the children dancing and frolicking on the stage. Emma's head slowly appeared above all the others. She waved again as she swivelled in her seat and half rose into a crouched position to face towards Rowdy.

Rowdy quickly eyed the entrance door that he had just passed through. Its opening provided an exit to safety and he was drawn to it by a force out of his control. The invisible drag towards the door only strengthened when he looked back towards Emma. She had returned to her seat but still had a hand raised. A mass of other heads now had their faces turned to look in Rowdy's direction, to see what the disturbance was all about. He had to fight the urge to make a quick dash for the door. Instead, he returned a little wave to his wife and others who were now watching. A forced smile teased the corners of his mouth.

He walked down the side aisle until reaching the row Emma was seated in. He entered the tightly packed horde and started to negotiate his way through the dense jungle of legs.

'Sorry,' he said softly to one lady, and removed his shoe from the top of her foot. The apologies kept flowing to every person he passed as he tripped over or kicked their legs. Some people made the effort to fold their legs to the side in an attempt to create more room for him to pass. Others hunched their knees upwards, but it was still like negotiating an obstacle course. Rowdy turned sideways to try and slimline his body as he shuffled along.

'Sorry,' he said to a woman sitting in the row in front as his backside collected the rear of her head, knocking her forward.

Rowdy finally made it to the vacant seat that Emma had reserved for him with her handbag. 'Is everything OK?' she whispered, leaning in close.

Not wanting to disturb the others around him, Rowdy leant towards Emma and softly replied, 'Yeah, fine.'

Emma tilted her head towards Rowdy and made the most of the loud applause as the children on stage finished their act. 'I saw you on the highway when I was bringing the kids up to Benstown. The accident didn't look too bad,' said Emma, recalling that she failed to see any apparent damage on the two vehicles that were stopped on the roadside.

Rowdy knew that sitting amongst three hundred other people was not the time to go into details and just replied, 'No, not too bad.'

Emma clapped along with the crowd of proud parents as the children on stage took a second bow. 'The kids would have been upset to think you weren't coming.'

'They would have survived,' replied Rowdy, somewhat harshly. 'Life's full of disappointments.'

The applause died away and the children disappeared into the side of the stage. The school principal, in his role as master of ceremonies, entered from the opposite side and announced, 'Ladies and gentleman, we will take a short break before our second half begins.'

The hall erupted as everyone in the audience started a conversation amongst themselves. The normal speaking level of people, when combined with hundreds resulted into an illegible cacophony. It was added to by the rumble a chair legs scrapping on the timber floor as people took the opportunity to stretch their legs or duck to the toilet.

Rowdy shrunk into his seat and did his best to look inconspicuous amongst the throng of people that totally overwhelmed him.

Dick had prepared the interview room in the same methodical manner he did most things. The tripod mounted video camera was placed in one corner of the room and ready to have its record button pushed. The single desk located in the small, box like room had been wiped over with disinfectant. Dick cleared the table of all non-essential items for the forensic procedure he was about to perform.

A sealed, clear plastic bag containing the mouth swab kit was placed in the centre of the table. Although the kit contained its own disposable gloves, Dick often found they would tear when putting them on, so he placed a box of latex gloves at one end of the table, but still within easy reach and view of the camera. The only other item on the desk was a small safety blade used to slice open the plastic packaging.

The suspect had been waiting patiently in the front foyer area after having the procedure explained to him by the continually moving and coffee-sipping Detective Sergeant Harker.

'Ahh Dick,' Detective Harker said as Dick appeared in the foyer area. 'Are you ready to go?'

'Just about. I want to confirm some details with you and Mr. Bell before I start.'

Dick took a couple of minutes to run through the circumstances of why and how the suspect Bell came to be at Brookstone Police Station to undergo a DNA swab. It was paramount that he made sure he was legally entitled to perform the forensic procedure. If he did not fulfil the legislative requirements, then evidence obtained from the DNA sample could be inadmissible in court and affect the whole outcome of a case.

Satisfied that Mr. Bell met all the criteria, Dick escorted him into the interview room and pushed record on the video camera.

It took Dick another ten minutes of reading through pages of legal jargon and ensuring Mr. Bell fully understood his rights and obligations before he could start the actual mouth swab procedure.

Dick sliced open the satchel and removed the contents. He made sure to keep his hands above the desk in full view of the camera while he slipped on a pair of gloves. He had seen, too often, police drop their hands down below the desk to apply their gloves out of view of the camera. Any defence barrister could later argue that while the officer's hands were out of sight, they could have contaminated them with DNA from the crime scene and then later transferred that DNA onto the mouth swab. Dick was overly careful and would give the defence no basis to mount an argument.

He was surprised when he found himself fumbling to open the sheath that sealed the sterile swab. At first he thought it was because of the ill-fitting gloves. Then he noticed his hands were shaking. It could not be from nerves, he had done this procedure hundreds of times. The more he concentrated on his hands, the worse they appeared to tremble. Not for the first time today he was again aware of the pounding in his head and the moisture starting to bead above his top lip.

Trying to ignore the beating in his chest, which was amplified to his ears, Dick continued on. Fortunately, the actual process of obtaining the swab takes less than a minute and was soon over when Dick pressed the twenty-cent piece sized moistened swab onto the sampling card. Dick cleared his throat before speaking again, afraid his voice would come out as a tortured squeak.

'Mr. Bell,' said Dick, as he started his last spiel to comply with the legislation and thankful there was some normality to its sound. 'Under the Act I am required to share your DNA sample with you so that you can have your DNA independently analysed and profiled should you wish to do so. I intend to share the material with you by allowing you to retain the swab. I have placed the swab back into the packet from which you originally obtained it and have sealed the packet with a barcode. This barcode has the same number as the barcode I will place on your consent form.'

Dick stopped the camera from recording. He couldn't explain it, but the apprehension and symptoms he was feeling seemed to stop at the same time.

7.00PM

The intermission at the school play had gone on longer than expected. Rowdy's eyes darted in every direction as he constantly scanned the crowd of people. He was not looking for anyone in particular, he was just continuing on from what he did at work every day. He was incapable of shutting out the packed hall that was buzzing with voices and just immersing himself in conversation with his wife. The discussion was totally one sided as Emma chatted away. Rowdy would manage a one word reply every so often as his concentration was focused on those people around him.

'Hey,' said Emma and placed a hand on Rowdy's leg and gave it an affectionate shake. 'I said the kids will be on next.'

His wife's touch momentarily caught his attention, but he still only managed to reply vacantly, 'Oh, that's good.'

While searching the faces in the room, Rowdy had also been listening to the loud tete-a-tete between the two women who sat directly in front of him. After a day where he had experienced death and the shattering of lives, the conversation between the two women grated on him as they discussed and whinged about the most trivial aspects of their lives. 'I think your hair looks fine,' said the chubby woman.

'I don't think the colour's right, though. It was the same colour as last time but done by a different girl and she just wasn't as good,' replied the obese woman.

The chubby woman made a start to say something but didn't manage a word when the obese woman continued. 'And look at the job they did on these nails,' she said while extending her fingers to show the other woman. 'I've a good mind to go back and ask for my money back.'

One of Rowdy's legs started to bounce on the ball of his foot as a release for the frustration that was building inside him. He restrained his urge to lean forward and tell the woman to get over it.

'I went to that new little coffee shop next to the hairdressers,' the obese woman said after barely taking a breath from her previous whine.

'How was it?' the smaller woman asked.

'Not very nice,' the obese woman replied, screwing up her pug nose. 'The coffee was dreadful. The service was slow and they didn't have a very large selection of tarts or slices to choose from.'

Rowdy physically bit his tongue as he could feel the insult concerning the woman's weight about to pass his lips.

'So you won't be going back there again?' asked the smaller round lady.

'I probably will. At least I don't have to walk far,'

'Lazy, fat, whinging bitch,' were the softly mumbled words uttered by Rowdy as both legs now bounced in agitation.

'What was that, dear?' Emma asked over the constant drone of noise that filled the hall which was now added to by the school band playing a tune.

'Nothing, just humming to the music,' replied Rowdy.

The obese woman's body hung in a roll of fat over the back of her seat. The chairs feeble legs visibly bowed each time she shifted her immense body. Rowdy's agitation was quelled somewhat as he imagined the woman collapsing to the floor as her chair folded beneath her under the strain. His hopes were not realised though as she continued her rant.

'I got this stupid checkout girl today who had no idea how to pack a shopping bag.'

'Some have no idea do they?' added the smaller woman.

'She mixed the frozen items in with the canned food. It was just a mess to unpack when I got home.'

The distraught and shattered image of Lynda Crisp returned to Rowdy. He could not imagine her complaining how her shopping bags were packed.

Rowdy's agitation found an instant cure the moment a troop of children filed onto the stage. The conversation between the two women ceased. The rumbling noise of the room soon subsided as everyone's attention returned to the stage.

Anne and Jordan stood without a hint of nerves, their faces beaming with excitement as the second play commenced. They moved confidently about the stage. Anne in her pretty frock and Jordan dressed as a pirate, complete with eye patch and stuffed parrot on his shoulder. Rowdy's own face mimicked his children's as he beamed with pride. Finally the day's events were locked away into a corner of his mind. He found a moment's peace as he marvelled at Emma's and his creations.

The calmness that he found in those fleeting moments was not to last. Soon the play would be over and Rowdy would be driving home with his children. The children would be talking excitedly about their day and Rowdy would try his hardest to concentrate and engage in their chatter. The images of his day would soon find their way out of the darkest corner and reappear in all their realism before his mind's eye. An unexplained remoteness would again consume him.

Dick secured the completed DNA sample kit into a refrigerator. First thing in the morning he would contact the couriers and organise it to be transported to the laboratory in Sydney to be analysed.

He was fixing the padlock on the fridge when Harker's voice echoed off the walls behind him. 'Thanks for that, Dick.'

'Anytime,' replied Dick as he rose from the small bar fridge and turned to face Garry.

'Look at the bright side of the coin,' said Garry, as he attempted to toss a positive spin on Dick's long day. 'If you're required to attend court, at least Coffs Harbour is a nice place to go on TA.'

Dick's lips spread into a smile but his eyes showed the fatigue that he was feeling. 'I'll go home and wax up the surfboard now,' he replied without enthusiasm.

'And if you need someone to carry your bags, I'm available,' added the detective, raising his coffee mug by way of a salute.

Dick gave an involuntary shudder at the thought of sharing a room with the Shrek look-a-like.

'I'll keep that in mind sarge,' replied Dick, and then added, 'Knowing you, I'm sure you'll weasel your way into the investigation and get a guernsey.'

Garry gave an exaggerated hurtful look that was soon replaced with a belly laugh that threatened to spill his coffee.

'I'm already working on it,' he finally managed to say.

The two officers parted and headed in opposite directions. Dick returned to his office and resumed the paperwork he had started nearly an hour ago.

'Just one more thing Dick,' said Harker as his head popped around Dick's doorway. 'Get a statement done for the swab ASAP.'

He did not bother to look up and continued leafing through some paperwork. He had already noted the statement preparation on his to do list. 'It's on the list,' replied Dick.

'Thanks again Dick,' and the sergeant's head disappeared.

Dick spent another twenty minutes at his desk to tidy up the necessary paperwork the day had created. The nonessential and less urgent entries still to be made would have to wait until tomorrow.

Just as he was finishing up, Dick's stomach growled to remind him how famished he was. He had not eaten since breakfast. He rose from his chair, stretched his heavy arms over his head and started towards the office door. It turned out he rose a little too quickly. On rounding the edge of his desk he had to pause for a moment as a dizzy spell caught him off balance. He placed a hand onto the desk to steady himself while blood slowly returned to his brain. He realised he was probably dehydrated as he also had not stopped to drink much during the day.

Once his balance returned and his vision cleared, Dick secured his firearm and made his way into the change room. With tremendous relief to his hips, he removed his appointment belt. He groaned with pleasure as the buckle unclipped and he let one side of the belt fall around his legs. He changed into his civilian clothes with the same routine that he had started the day.

Dick checked the time. It was after seven-thirty and the sun had rested long ago. Only three hours late leaving tonight, he thought positively. Just as he was about to take his first steps towards the door, his mobile phone rang. He placed a hand on his pocket as if trying to smother the ring tone. He was tempted not to answer it. Just go home he told himself. It is never good news.

Dick sighed as he found himself removing the phone from his pocket. 'Hello,' he said in a voice that disguised his fatigue.

'Dick, Rob Cooley,' greeted the Inspector from the other end of a telephone up on the first floor of the building.

'Hi, boss,' Dick said with a heavy voice. 'What can I do for you?'

'Nothing at all. I was just talking with Garry Harker. He said you were still in the building,' said the Duty Officer.

'I'm just about to walk out the door as we speak,' said Dick, making his way down the hallway towards the rear exit of the police station.

'I won't hold you up. Just wanted to tell you I have sent an email to the Healthy Lifestyles Branch about the accident today. It was a nasty one,' stated the Duty Officer.

'I suppose it was,' replied Dick.

'Anyway,' continued the Duty Officer, 'I've also contacted the EAP to organise a debrief.'

The Employee Assistance Programme was outsourced to provide psychological counselling and was available to all police in the state on an individual basis. 'Righto,' replied Dick, too tired to argue. 'They know where to find me.'

'I'll keep you posted when I know more,' said the Duty Officer before terminating the call.

Dick returned the phone to his pocket. He reached out and turned the handle on the exit door and swung it inwards. A voice, filled with urgency, jolted Dick as it boomed from a speaker fitted into the ceiling above his head. The wail of a siren competed with the voice for the radio operator's attention.

Dick stood frozen in the doorway as he immediately recognised the officer's voice calling the start of a pursuit. Dick was immediately taken back deep into his past. It was not just his hands shaking this time. His whole body shook as he listened to the pursuit unfold. His stomach knotted but not from hunger cravings.

'Don't do it,' Dick said aloud. 'Call it off, Phantom.' Dick's voice quivered as he spoke.

The pursuit continued to be called over the airway. With renewed strength and a deep timber to his voice, Dick looked up and forcibly said to the speaker as if using it as a direct connection to the driver calling the pursuit. *Terminate now!*

*****

EPILOGUE

Ricky bounced up the stairs two at a time to the first floor office. The thick woollen carpet under his feet, which still had that new smell to it, acted like a springboard to his already agile and youthful exuberance. The weighty gun belt around his middle did not encumber his movements in any way.

It was the first time Ricky had been in a psychiatrist's office. He slowed his ascent back to one step at a time as he neared the large, open entrance platform of the doctor's waiting room. His foot landed slowly off the last step onto the floor level. His head swivelled and his eyes darted around the waiting room. He was not sure what to expect, but it certainly was not the fresh uncluttered room that greeted him.

Directly in front of him was a long, chest-high reception desk that curved to create a semicircle work area behind. Its front façade was a decorative pattern of coloured laminates. The colours blended like an artist's palette from sandy beige to a bluish-green aquamarine then merged at its horizon into an azure blue.

The wall behind the reception desk was one large pane of glass from floor to ceiling. Its vertical blinds were completely drawn back to either side. The glass was spotless to the point it appeared invisible. It gave the impression you could walk straight through onto the beach and dive into the ocean that lay beyond. Ricky then realised that the reception desk was the abstract representation of the view framed by the window behind it.

The pastel walls of the room were brought to life with vibrant paintworks depicting the Amalfi coast and Greek islands in the Mediterranean. One painting was so large, Ricky could almost step aboard the yacht depicted and sail the crystal clear waters.

A fish tank was built into another wall. Bright tropical fish swam its three metre length. Their scales sparkled as the harsh fluorescent lighting played along their flanks. A mesmerising affect soon blanketed Ricky as he watched their graceful movements.

A sense of calm filled him as he approached the reception desk. A spectacled, dark haired woman came into view as Ricky moved closer. The reflection of the computer monitor in front of her danced across her glasses as she typed. The words that streamed across the screen appeared only an instant after they were spoken into her headphones from the Dictaphone to which they were connected. A smiling face looked up and greeted Ricky as he placed his forearms flat on the marble counter top.

'Good morning,' said the smiling face. The receptionist lifted a headphone earpiece and rested it above her ear. Before Ricky could return the greeting, the pleasant lady continued, 'Please take a seat. Doctor Larbrashski won't be long.'

'Thank-you,' replied Ricky politely.

He thought it odd the receptionist did not ask to confirm his name and appointment. Then he considered that with hour long appointments, he should not have expected a full waiting room.

Ricky sank into a plush chair under a painting of a Sorrento coastline. The Italian artists name that appeared in the bottom right corner meant nothing to Ricky. He lounged back into his chair and studied the spectacular ocean view through the window, thankful that he was not paying for all this.

No sooner had Ricky taken his seat; another police officer appeared at the top of the stairwell and entered the waiting room. Rowdy walked straight up to the reception desk past Ricky without even a glance in his direction.

Ricky was impressed how well turned out the other officer was. He noticed the crisp uniform with knife edge creases lining the sleeves of his police shirt. The same could be seen running down the centre of his trousers. The officer's glistening, black appointment belt matched the spit-shine he had to his boots. Rowdy crossed the room in front of Ricky. His shoulders were pinned back and his posture upright in military fashion.

Rowdy had a brief conversation with the receptionist, and then turned away. As he walked around the small coffee table in the centre of the room he paused to shuffle through the assortment of reading material that it contained. Rowdy passed by the car magazines and settled on a luxury boat magazine instead.

Ricky thought he noticed a slight nod of the head in acknowledgement towards him by the other officer as he approached with his magazine in hand. Ricky returned the gesture.

Rowdy checked the bright red cushioned chair for any signs of its previous occupant before lowering himself into it. The whole room was spotless and there was no need to brush crumbs or any other foreign matter from the seat.

He made himself comfortable, crossed a leg over one knee and started to flick through the magazine.

His ability to concentrate was getting worse and no matter how hard he tried to read an article, he found himself constantly having to read back over what he read, several times, in order to comprehend it. Instead he looked at the pictures and placed himself on board the luxury cruisers, trying to smell the sea air and feel the salt spray on his face.

Dick's forty-two year old arthritic hips protested their way to the top of the stairs by stabbing him with short sharp jabs like a knife. The discomfort lessened now he walked across the soft level floor towards the reception desk and repositioned his gun belt.

'Hello, Dick,' said the receptionist, followed by a warm smile.

'Hi, Mandy,' replied Dick, flashing a smile. 'How are you?'

'You know me, too busy to be anything but fine,' she replied happily.

Dick pointed towards the view behind her, 'And so you should be, working with a view like that.'

The receptionist swivelled her chair and took in the ocean scene through the expanse of glass. 'I'm too busy to even notice it half the time,' she said.

'What a waste,' said Dick when she swivelled back to face him.

The receptionist reached up with her left hand and placed it on the headphone earpiece resting on the side of her head. 'Doctor won't be long,' she said as she refitted the headphone into place over her ear, to let Dick know the conversation was over, and returned to her work.

Dick headed straight to the water cooler and filled a small plastic cup. Careful not to spill any of its contents, he managed to manoeuvre his aching joints into the comfort of a waiting chair. The police officer he sat next to did not look up from the magazine he appeared to be reading.

The young police officer sat tapping his hands on his thighs as the impatience of waiting mounted. Dick noticed that every twentieth beat or so , the young constable checked his wrist watch. He sat patiently, sipping his water, enjoying the view and wondered how great it would be to have the energy again to drum his thighs.

A second row of identical waiting-chairs lined the wall adjoining the three police officers. Sitting in a chair nearest the reception desk, and with a view that could encompass the entire room towards the stairwell, was a man. He had been patiently sitting, but somewhat nervously, and watching intently as the three police officers entered the room. None of the officers appeared to look at him. Perhaps he just blended into the pastel coloured wall and did not stand out as attention was drawn to the colourful fish tank built into the wall at which he sat. No matter. The more he blended in, the better he felt.

The man sat with his knees together. His hands, marked by age, lay in his lap and unconsciously rubbed together as if he was washing them. His shoulders slumped as if carrying an enormous burden. At forty-five years of age, he was not much older than the last policeman he had watched come in.

His facial features told a lie, though. His forehead was furrowed into a constant frown, causing his eyebrows to lower and shade his eyes into a look of displeasure, or was it deep concentration. The crow-feet lines that bordered his eyes pushed them into a permanent squint which emphasised the puffy bags under them. They were like pillows for the sadness in his eyes to rest on. The dark rings that hung in the creases below, clearly told the story of a man who had witnessed too much of the wrong side of life and all its hardships.

The man appeared fifteen years older than his age suggested. He sat exhausted, both physically and emotionally, as if his life was already spent. His self-esteem drained. Broken was the will to fight the helplessness that absorbed him. He starred vacantly at the three strangers through eyes that could no longer distinguish the past from the present.

'Doctor Larbrashski will see you now,' said the receptionist, her head popping above the marbled counter top.

Ricky, Rowdy and Dick all rose to their feet in unison. Ricky made his way to the closed door with a brass name plate affixed to it. Rowdy leant towards the coffee table and tossed his magazine onto the pile of others. Dick dropped his empty cup into a garbage bin beside the water cooler as he passed.

Ricky placed his hand onto the door knob. Rowdy and Dick stood behind him in single file. Ricky looked down at his hand as he began to turn the handle. The taut, unmarked, youthful skin on the back of his hand dissolved away as it turned the handle further. It was replaced with the dried creased skin of a much older man. Damaged, by years of exposure to the sun, it had the dull weathered look of timber that had lost its coat of paint.

The door was pushed ajar.

Doctor Larbrashski sat behind his large timber desk, reviewing the file of his next patient. In contrast to the brightness of the waiting room, his office was dimly lit. Blinds were partially drawn and the sconce lighting gave off a yellowish glow that was absorbed by dark timber panelled walls.

The room was decorated with a nautical theme and anyone entering for the first time felt they just entered the Captain's cabin on a seventeenth century Man O' War. Far from being dull and dreary, the room achieved the same calming ambience as the waiting room. It had a cosy feel which was perfect for a one-on-one consultation.

Doctor Larbrashski ran a finger down the page as he scanned the covering sheet of the file which read:-

Patient: - Richard Alexander McCrae
Occupation: - Former Police Officer
Discharged on medical grounds
Medical Condition: - Post Traumatic Stress Disorder

Significant Events: - Too numerous to recount individually
Brief summary between 1986 - 2007
- *Fatal high speed pursuit*
- *Numerous deceased persons involving putridity*
- *Numerous deceased persons involving dismemberment*
- *Numerous deceased persons by hanging*
- *Numerous deceased persons by gun shot*
- *Numerous deceased persons involving infants and children*
- *Numerous deceased persons by fire*
- *Numerous deceased persons, decapitation involved*
- *Numerous deceased persons by drowning*
- *Numerous fatal and serious motor vehicle collisions*

The psychiatrist looked up from his folder as the door opened. The outline of a man was silhouetted by the stark bright light that shone behind him from the waiting room. As the door closed behind him and he made his way out of the gloom towards the single studded leather chair that waited at the front of the doctor's desk, the man's features became distinguishable.

The inconspicuous man had sat patiently in the waiting room, absorbed in visions and recollections of his past.

When he entered the doctor's office, he left behind at the door the three strangers that he held some vague recognition of, perhaps from another life. Surely it was not him that had done those things. It must have been someone else.

He sank meekly into the chair. The leather creaked stiffly under his weight as he organised his stiffened joints into some degree of comfort. The man had grown out of Ricky long ago. Rowdy just seemed incongruous these days. His christened name of Richard seemed too aristocratic to be attached to the fragile shell of a man who struggled to clean toilets for a living. He preferred the abbreviated form of his name most.

'So Dick,' the psychiatrist said with a warm inviting voice. 'How are you today?'

Dick did not reply immediately. A faint ember of spark still managed to break through his sullen, deep brown eyes as pride filled his worn features with life.

'Fine Doc,' Dick replied, still refusing to give into his demons. 'Just getting through another day.'

*****